WITHDRAWN
UTSA LIBRARIES

D1601336

Strategic Planning in Healthcare

Building a Quality-Based Plan Step by Step

Bernard J. Horak, Ph.D.

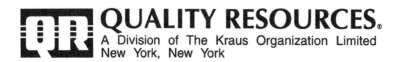

QUALITY RESOURCES.
A Division of The Kraus Organization Limited
New York, New York

Most Quality Resources books are available at quantity discounts when purchased in bulk. more information contact:

Special Sales Department
Quality Resources
A Division of the Kraus Organization Limited
902 Broadway
New York, New York 10010
800-247-8519
212-979-8600

Copyright 1997 Bernard J. Horak, Ph.D.

All right reserved. No part of this work covered by the copyrights hereon may be reproduce or used in any form or by any means—graphic, electronic, or mechanical, including photocopying, recording, taping, or information storage and retrieval systems—without written permission of the publisher.

Printed in the United States of America

01 00 99 98 97   10 9 8 7 6 5 4 3 2 1

The paper used in this publication meets the minimum requirements of American National Standard for Information Sciences—Permanence of Paper for Printed Library Materials, Al Z39.48-1984.

ISBN 0-527-76314-4

Library of Congress Cataloging-in-Publication Data
Horak, Bernard J.
    Strategic planning in healthcare: building a quality-based plan step-by-step / Berna J. Horak.
        p.   cm.
    Includes bibliographical references and index.
    ISBN 0-527-76314-4 (alk. paper)
    1. Health services administration. 2. Strategic planning. 3. Total quality managemer 4. Medical care—Quality control. I. Title.
RA971.H577 1997
362.1'068—dc21   96-53418
                                       CIP

DEDICATION

This book is dedicated to my children:
Rachel, David, Molly, and Willy

I love you all very much and now will have more time
to spend with you.

TABLE OF CONTENTS

LIST OF FIGURES

LIST OF TABLES

PREFACE

The origins of this book can be traced back to my experience as the director of strategic planning and total quality management at Walter Reed Army Medical Center. In this position I had the tremendous opportunity of integrating two vital functions of organizational change.

The vision for this integration was established by the medical center commander, Major General Richard Cameron, M.D., and Colonel Joan Zajtchuk, M.D., who was director of clinical services and my direct supervisor. These two individuals envisioned the benefits of more focused change, the linking of quality improvement projects to strategic initiatives, and the potential for TQM principles to enhance the strategic planning process. The most powerful principles were the emphasis on the customer, the use of interdisciplinary teams, training, and the playing of "catch-ball" across the organization. It was found that these resulted in increased acceptance or buy-in, the integration of department plans, and a far better strategic plan for the organization. Additionally, it was felt that the philosophy of continuous improvement made Walter Reed more responsive to patient and staff needs and prevented the strategic plan (and the resulting department plans) from collecting dust on the shelf.

The benefits were not easily realized. A considerable amount of learning and redirection of efforts had to take place. Fortunately, we took note of these activities and lessons.

After accepting a teaching position at The George Washington University (GWU), I began to reflect on and synthesize this experience with that of other healthcare and non-healthcare organizations. My learning found its way into the introductory course, Health Services Planning and Marketing and the advance course, Strategic Planning in the Department of Health Services Management and Policy. I have also had the opportunity to speak and consult on the topic of quality-based strategic planning. These opportunities, particularly feedback after each engagement, further developed my understanding of what works (or doesn't work) in healthcare organizations.

The two most important things I learned from these experiences were the use of the clinical model (assessment–planning–implementation–evaluation) and the criticality of the implementation phase of the model. Both are incorporated in this book. The clinical model becomes my basic framework for strategic planning and a chapter is devoted to implementation.

Finally, the actual process of writing this book resulted in additional refinement of my ideas and approach to strategic planning. This caused me to further develop and organize my thoughts and experiences. Most beneficial were the comments by the editors at Quality Resources, particularly Cindy Tokumitsu, and by the anonymous reviewers. Probably the most beneficial suggestion was from a reviewer who recommended that I synthesize the various strategies and approaches. The result was the "Roadmap"—a step-by-step guide that the reader can use as a starting point for his or her own organization.

ACKNOWLEDGMENTS

This book would not have been possible without the support of my family. The importance of their understanding with regards to time and getting me through frequent bouts of writer's block cannot be overstated.

I also wish to thank Dr. Richard S. Southby, my mentor and the chair of the Department of Health Services Management and Policy at The George Washington University, for his support and encouragement as I completed the book.

Additionally, I wish to thank the many organizations that have provided me information and case examples. In particular, I wish to acknowledge the following for opening up their organization to contribute to this project:

Optima Health, Inc., Manchester, New Hampshire (Bob Chilotte, CEO; Phil Ryan, president; Mary Ann Eldred, director of non-acute services and TQM; Dr. Stephen Tzianabos, medical director; and Denise Place, director of quality and utilization management).

Walter Reed Army Medical Center, Washington, D.C. (Major General Ronald R. Blanck, M.D., commander; Major General Richard Cameron, M.D., former commander; Colonel Joan Zajtchuk, M.D., former deputy for clinical services; and Les Howell, director of performance improvement).

Sisters of Charity Health Care System (Gayle Capozzalo, senior vice president–strategic development).

Finally, I thank my editor, Maggie Pierson; my editor at Quality Resources, Cindy Tokumitsu; and the manuscript reviewers who provided valuable advice and input.

CHAPTER 1

INTRODUCING QUALITY-BASED STRATEGIC PLANNING

✓ *"If a society aims for quality, rewards quality, discusses quality, devises ways of measuring and monitoring quality, takes determined and effective actions to restore any absence of quality, identifies itself openly and constantly with quality, it will almost certainly get quality."*

—National Association for Healthcare Quality

✓ *"The fundamental change that is needed (by American companies) is that quality is adopted as a business strategy. This strategy is applicable to all types of organizations."*

—Nolan

"One of the most difficult challenges faced by any senior executive is how to turn strategy into action."

—Anonymous

Quality improvement is now a major area of strategic interest for healthcare organizations. Quality-based strategic planning ensures that the organization is attractive to its major stakeholders or customers: patients, employees, physicians, third party payers, and the community at large. Clearly, an effective quality strategy can result in a distinct competitive advantage when coupled with other strategic thrusts, particularly cost reduction and customer satisfaction.

This book offers a basic framework for quality-based strategic planning (QBSP) through a model based on experience and an analysis of literature in the areas of strategic planning and quality improvement. The framework gives managers an approach to move simultaneously with quality, cost, and customer satisfaction initiatives.

Using this framework, the book discusses case examples in which QBSP was applied in healthcare organizations, including a detailed case study in which this author served as director of strategic planning and total quality management (TQM). The book concludes with a discussion of lessons learned and implications for further application of QBSP in healthcare organizations. The book also provides specific tools the manager can use to implement a quality strategy— "to turn strategy into action."

Quality-Based Strategic Planning— An Overview

Quality-based strategic planning works best when quality planning is fully integrated with the strategic planning process. The ultimate result is one strategic plan which incorporates quality goals and includes total quality management philosophy in the development of objectives, action plans, and mission, vision, and value statements.

To stakeholders, the strategic plan will show a long-term commitment to quality initiatives and a quality philosophy embedded in all organizational objectives.

The basic tenets of QBSP include the use of a systems approach and employee and management involvement at all levels. The process essentially consists of an assessment of stakeholder/customer needs and expectations, identification of goals and specific actions to meet those needs and expectations, implementation of changes, and continuous measurement, follow-up, and improvement. Thus, QBSP can be defined as an organization-wide, systematic, and customer-focused process to reach the long-term quality goals of the organization.

The Integration of Strategic Planning and TQM

QBSP integrates planning and total quality management (TQM). It uses the existing strategic planning process of assessing market and organizational needs, developing vision and mission statements, determining goals and priorities, and allocating resources to goals/priorities. The underlying philosophy and approaches of quality improvement are applied to the strategic planning process. These quality improvement concepts include customer focus, empowerment, systems approach, measurement, and continuous improvement.

By judiciously integrating TQM into strategic planning, you avoid the common pitfalls often found when each is implemented in isolation. Implementing TQM without strategic planning can result in the following:

1. Not having a focus or a sense of direction for the quality effort, resulting in projects which are not linked to the strategic goals of the organization.

2. Taking limited, operational view of improvements, thus relying on measures of progress such as reductions in cycle times or defect rates. While these are important efforts, they may not provide the competitive advantage in times of changing markets, customer preferences, and technologies ("Beyond Total Quality Management," 1995).

3. Working on improving processes which are in transition, about to be eliminated, or add little organizational value. Says Sir Royce (in Tally, 1991, p.31): "There is nothing more wasteful than doing efficiently that which is not necessary."

4. Not having a total systems view, resulting in treating processes as unconnected islands, thus failing to consider the interaction and effects upon all processes and organizational systems when redesigning or improving an existing process ("Beyond Total Quality Management," 1995).

5. Focusing on the "quick fix"—devoting efforts to fire-fighting and immediate problems rather than to opportunities and long-term solutions.

6. Not having organizational support and commitment for quality improvement or quality management since quality initiatives are not included in the strategic plan.

On the other hand, drawbacks of implementing strategic planning without TQM include:

1. Planning being directed in a top-down manner by senior managers and planners, resulting in a lack of understanding and acceptance of organizational goals and priorities by middle management and the rank and file.

2. Planning being viewed as a one-time event, repeated every few years or when the capital budget is prepared. Thus, plans often collect dust because of a lack of continuous review and update.

3. Not having outcome measures to determine the effectiveness of the goals.

4. Not including quality-related goals due to an emphasis on cost reduction and immediate operational demands.

5. Planning which is not integrated and coordinated across departments if the planning process consisted of the "roll-up" of individual departments' plans. This results in suboptimization and lack of focus on organization-wide needs.

Critical Elements of Quality-Based Strategic Planning

Below are the critical elements of QBSP. These are synthesized from the work of multiple sources and authorities in the areas of strategic planning and quality improvement. Among these are Juran, Deming, the Joint Commission on Accreditation of Healthcare Organizations (JCAHO), the Malcolm Baldrige National Quality Award Criteria, and the experience of the author and others who have successfully utilized QBSP concepts. The elements are more fully discussed in the text through the use of case studies and examples to illustrate how these concepts and various related tools can be applied.

Quality as a Strategic Imperative

Quality must be made a strategic imperative. This means that specific quality goals must be included in the strategic plan and that quality improvement activities are integrated into the strategic planning process. Goals are set that focus the organization's quality efforts on meeting or exceeding customer needs and on improving processes designed to meet these needs. The result will be "doing the right thing" and "doing the right thing well"—JCAHO's two dimensions of performance.

Constancy of Purpose

Constancy of purpose, the first of Deming's fourteen points to quality (see Table 1.1), consists of three parts: (1) a vision statement of where the organization wants to be; (2) a mission statement of the needs and expectations that the organization intends to fulfill; and (3) a set of beliefs, values, or guiding principles that define how the mission will be accomplished. Developing these three elements is the first step in the QBSP process, setting the tone and providing the direction for the development of quality goals across the organization.

Table 1.1: Deming's Fourteen Points

1. Create constancy of purpose for the improvement of product and service.
2. Adopt the new philosophy.
3. Cease dependence on mass inspection.
4. End the practice of awarding business on price tag alone.
5. Improve constantly and forever the system of production and service.
6. Institute training and retraining.
7. Institute leadership.
8. Drive out fear.
9. Break down barriers between staff areas.
10. Eliminate slogans, exhortations, and targets for the workforce.
11. Eliminate numerical quotas.
12. Remove barriers to pride of workmanship.
13. Institute a vigorous program of education and retraining.
14. Take action to accomplish the transformation.

Customer Focus

Being "customer-focused" means designing and providing services which meet or exceed the needs and expectations of customers—patients, third-party payers, and the community. This is usually accomplished via the planning tools of market/customer research through the use of focus groups, demographic analysis, and community health assessments. The need and benefit of a customer-focused approach was well stated by one member of an implementation planning team at the SSM Health Care System (Capozzalo, 1993, p. 18):

> When we used to do strategic planning, we'd say,
> "I have $3 million, how do I spend it?"
> Today, we ask, "How do I determine and meet
> the needs of my community and my customers,
> and what dollars will it take to do that?"

An excellent customer-first model is Juran's "Quality Planning Roadmap," which consists of the identification of customers, the determination of customers' needs and expectations, and the design (or redesign) of products and services to meet those needs and expectations.

The concept of customer focus also applies to internal customers. Thus, the needs and expectations of external customers must be reconciled with those of employees, physicians, and vendors/contractors. These needs and expectations are identified through such means as surveys, focus groups, interviews with physicians, and "town-hall" type meetings with employees.

Systems Approach

An organization is a system—an interdependent set of organizational parts with a common purpose. Unfortunately, healthcare organizations (HCOs) are often organized as a disconnected collection of departments and services. As mentioned earlier, this results in suboptimization—departments functioning without regard for what is best for the entire organization. The JCAHO has recognized that the organization must operate as a system and has required that all department directors show how their departments contribute to the hospital's primary functions and how they are coordinating and integrating services and activities.

Quality Culture

If necessary, a cultural change must be made so that the organization's mission, goals, and values are understood and internalized by managers and employees. The ultimate aim is to convert the hospital into one that is dedicated to quality—one in which quality planning and improvement becomes a part of the day-to-day operations. This occurs through such actions as:

- Top management commitment: providing necessary resources, role modeling of desired behaviors, and rewarding and recognizing staff for efforts in improving quality.

- Operationalizing the value statements through an in-depth orientation program and education on how the values can be applied in the work setting.

- Providing training in principles and tools of quality improvement. These tools include a structured problem-solving approach, team-building, and the use of statistics, flow charts, and cause-effect diagrams.

- Empowering managers and employees with the authority to address problems at the lowest possible level and by the playing of "catch-ball"—the sharing and receiving of input on organizational goals.

Structure

An organizational structure is needed to oversee QBSP efforts. Usually this takes the form of a steering council (SC), which has authority and represents all major parts of the organization. Their missions are to define the strategic planning process; recommend strategic quality plans and organization-wide performance measures; charter quality projects and cross-functional quality teams; coordinate efforts across departments and teams; and review the effectiveness of all quality plans.

Internal Assessment

In order to insure that the organization reaches its goals, it must remove organizational barriers (things that get in the way of quality) and identify its strengths (things that the organization can use or rely on as it moves towards its goals). This is part of the SWOT (strengths, weaknesses, opportunities, and threats) analysis of the planning assessment. Among variables examined would be employee morale, medical staff involvement, skills in quality planning and improvement, structure, organizational resources allocated to quality, and the degree of commitment by leaders.

Two excellent models for internal quality assessments are the Malcolm Baldrige Award National Quality Award Criteria and the JCAHO Guidelines for Improving Organization Performance.

Measurement and Analysis

Evaluation must be made on how well the organization is meeting its goals and the needs and expectations of its customers. Data should be used at every level of the organization and the data must be timely, reliable, and valid. Methods for analysis include statistical process control, benchmarks, surveys of patient satisfaction, and clinical outcome standards.

Continuous Improvement

Regardless of the success of plans, an organization should never relax. It must constantly seek out opportunities and maintain an attitude of an unrelenting quest for improvement. In addition, JCAHO requires that every HCO have a performance improvement model. The two most effective and common models are the Shewhart Cycle (Plan-Do-Check-Act) and the Action Research/Organization Development Model (Assessment, Planning, Implementation, and Evaluation). Aggressive implementation of such frameworks will increase the likelihood that changes will be sustained over the long term.

A Model for Quality-Based Strategic Planning

Figure 1.1 outlines a model for QBSP which serves as the framework for discussions in the succeeding chapters. As seen, the model is based on the organization development model of assessment, planning, implementation, and evaluation. This model is also consistent with the existing framework of clinical practice which includes the same four phases. The model incorporates all nine elements described previously and is based on the experience of the author.

The discussion below provides the basic approach to the model and a description of two other approaches sometimes taken by organizations. The chapter concludes with an overview of the model's four phases.

Basic Approach

The model has, as its basis, the strategic planning process found in most healthcare organizations. By integrating

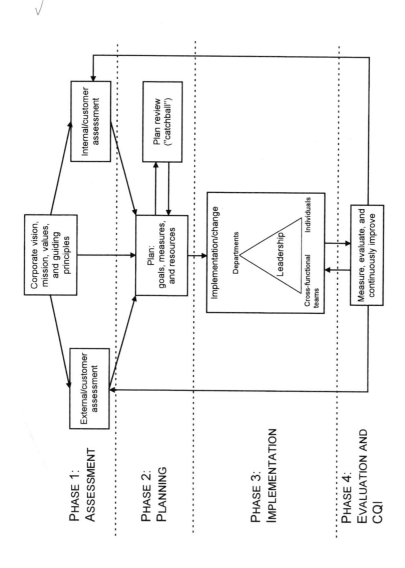

Figure 1.1 Model for Quality-Based Strategic Planning

quality improvement into the strategic planning process, quality goals are developed in conjunction with other organizational goals, such as financial performance, capital improvement, market share, mergers, and affiliations. Hence, quality improvement becomes a strategic imperative and plans are put in place to "make quality happen."

Additionally, in an integrated approach, all strategic initiatives are planned with quality concepts in mind. Thus, strategic planning becomes more robust and effective through the application of such concepts as empowerment, customer focus, and data measurement. The integration also means that quality initiatives are based on an assessment of market conditions and reflect organizational priorities. This greatly facilitates organizational support in terms of leadership commitment and resources to quality improvement efforts.

Under QBSP model, one steering council serves for both strategic planning and quality improvement. This council usually consists of the CEO and selected members of the senior management team (for example, the COO and VPs of the medical staff, finance, planning, human resources, and quality). The council determines the corporate vision, mission, values, and guiding principles for the organization. Experience reveals that dual councils for planning and quality improvement provide confusion, waste valuable executive time, and slow quality efforts.

To start up and monitor quality initiatives, a "working group" or "resource group" is usually designated by the steering council. This group assists in such areas as analyzing assessments of customer needs and expectations and recommending quality indicators, improvement priorities, and process improvement teams. Nevertheless, all activity is coordinated and approved by the steering council.

Other Approaches

Two other approaches to QBSP are often found in organizations. However, these approaches do not involve the full integration of quality and strategic planning.

The first involves quality planning conducted by a separate quality council (QC). The QC takes its cues from the strategic plan or top executives. Thus, it usually accepts the vision, mission, organizational values, guiding principles, and strategic imperatives as given. From these, the QC develops a roll-out plan.

The other approach basically involves the use of quality improvement techniques in strategic planning. Unfortunately, this usually consists of no more than "borrowing" facilitators from the quality staff to conduct strategic planning sessions in which such tools as brainstorming, force-field analysis, or nominal group techniques are used to develop organizational goals. These goals may not necessarily be in areas of quality improvement.

Overview of the Model

The following discussion provides a description of the integrated approach to strategic planning and quality improvement. As mentioned previously, it follows the familiar framework of the clinical model of assessment, planning, implementation, and evaluation.

Phase 1: Assessment

The QBSP process always begins with a review of the development of vision, mission, and organizational values/guiding principles. These areas not only guide what is important during the assessment phase, but moreover, provide the overarching umbrella for all organizational planning and action. Additionally, they can become guides for decision making and behavior for all managers and the workforce, thereby precluding the need for lengthy policy and procedure manuals.

The external assessment examines variables in the external environment that may affect quality, such as technology, regulation, and the availability of skilled employees. Additionally, the healthcare organization (HCO) identifies and analyzes the needs and expectations of its external customers which include patients, families, third-party payers, and the community at large.

The internal assessment looks at organizational strengths and weaknesses, particularly barriers to quality improvement and the environment or culture for quality initiatives. The internal assessment also consists of an evaluation of the needs and expectations of internal customers (employees, physicians, and the board of directors).

Phase 2: Planning

The planning phase is the most involved. It is here that the steering council takes the input from the internal and external assessments and considers options in light of the vision, mission, and values/guiding principles. Through such techniques as gap analysis and benchmarking, the SC formulates goals, objectives, and strategies to reach each objective. Additionally, action plans which include resource requirements, time frames for completion, and internal benchmarks (or measures for success) are developed. These plans are then shared with managers at all levels to obtain their input before a final strategic quality plan is published.

Phase 3: Implementation

Implementation is truly the hard part—the phase in which plans either succeed or fail. It requires close attention to the assessment of organizational culture, particularly barriers to, and leverage points for, change.

The key to implementation is leadership. Leaders need a profound understanding of quality concepts and a commitment to the QBSP process which they must be able to demonstrate convincingly. Managers need to view quality improvement as "their business" and not a program run by the quality staff.

There are three other major areas of focus during implementation. The first is the existing structure of departments and services (e.g., medicine, surgery, psychiatry, orthopedics, pharmacy, admitting). The strategic quality goals of the organization must be operationalized and efforts undertaken to identify and conduct improvement initiatives specific to each department or service.

Another area of focus is the establishment and use of cross-functional teams. The teams are necessary since most process improvement initiatives extend past department and service lines. Cross-functional teams are chartered by the steering council and trained as a team in quality and process improvement.

The final area focuses on individual employees. To empower employees, all should be given training in the basic concepts of quality improvement—particularly their role as a supplier of service to patients and fellow employees.

Leaders must set the tone, model behaviors, and provide incentives to create a working environment in which quality improvement is everyone's job.

Phase 4: Evaluation and Continuous Quality Improvement

Phase 4 facilitates continuous improvement by measuring and analyzing the results of the plan and its implementation. Most helpful during this phase are the benchmarks or measures of success which were established in Phase 2. The reasons for not meeting benchmarks are carefully studied. Based on this analysis and on new external and internal assessments, plans are revised and new actions put in place for change.

QBSP never ends. As stated by David Kearns, former CEO of Xerox, "Quality is a race without a finish line." (Schmidt & Finnigan, 1992). The term "continuous quality improvement," or CQI, is used to refer to the unrelenting drive for enhancement of clinical and administrative services. The QBSP model, with its four interrelated phases, is an iterative process that better ensures that CQI happens for the benefit of all the customers of the healthcare organization.

Organization of the Book

Each of the next four chapters examines a phase of the model using the following:

1. Relevant concepts or elements.

2. Various techniques or tools which can be utilized.

3. Examples of how the concepts and tools are applied.

4. A summary in the form of a "roadmap"—an outline of the key tasks and activities for managers to consider. This roadmap integrates information from various case studies and examples.

Chapter 6 discusses current issues, including quality improvement during times of mergers, acquisitions, and cost containment. Chapter 7 provides three detailed case studies of QBSP. Chapter 8 discusses conclusions and lessons learned from the cases, the literature, and experience of the writer.

CHAPTER 2

ASSESSMENT

Quality-based strategic planning starts with the formulation or modification of statements of mission, vision, and operating principles. Quality concepts must be integrated into these documents and these concepts must be understood by managers and employees at all levels.

Six crucial questions must be answered during the assessment, the first phase of strategic quality planning:

1. What is our mission and vision?
2. What are our operating principles or values as we pursue our mission and vision?
3. Who are our stakeholders?
4. What are their needs and expectations?
5. What are the variables in the external environment (particularly threats and opportunities) which must be considered?
6. What are our internal strengths and weaknesses?

The Mission

Mission statements provide the purposes for organization, answering questions of identity. An example of a mission statement follows:

17

Community Hospital Association is a not-for-profit corporation. Its mission and the purposes for which the corporation is formed are:

1. *To establish, maintain, and operate hospitals.*
2. *To carry on educational activities related to the care of the sick and injured, or promotion of health.*
3. *To promote and carry on scientific research related to care of the sick and injured, or promotion of health.*
4. *To engage in any activity designed to promote the general health of the community.*

Other examples of mission statements, as well as statements of vision and guiding principles or values, are found in Appendix A. As one can see, these statements often overlap or are merged into one document. All are intended, however, to provide direction for the organization.

The Vision and Guiding Principles/Values

The vision statement is a description of what the HCO should be at some future point in time. It is the capstone of any strategy, setting the future direction for the organization. If the vision is communicated and understood by the HCO's stakeholders, particularly its employees, it can be a powerful force for obtaining commitment to organizational goals. Vision statements need not be lengthy; they can be simple, but effective, as in the following examples:

- To be the pediatric hospital of choice on the East Coast.
- To be the healthcare organization that is most highly regarded for its commitment to patients, payers, and employees.

As seen in Appendix A, vision or mission statements often include organizational philosophy or beliefs (e.g., "commitment to employees," "customer friendliness," "continual improvement of services"). Usually, these are termed guiding principles or organizational values.

These principles remain constant, whereas vision and mission statements change on the basis of environmental or market conditions. Thus, the principles give stability and constancy of purpose to the organization. Charles B. Van Vorst, president and CEO of the Mercy Health Care Corporation and the Mercy Hospital and Medical Center in Chicago, has said, "Our employees need something to hold on to—to ground my people—with all the organizational changes which are going on around them."

Principles and values also provide the guidance for organizational management decision making and strategy. As stated by Walt Disney, "The decisions are easy if you know what your values are."

Additionally, principles and values statements can become behavioral guides for all managers and employees, thereby precluding the need for lengthy policy or procedure manuals and close supervision. Thus, principles and values provide a prime vehicle for employee empowerment—a concept now strongly espoused for its motivational and organizational benefits.

The following is a value statement from Darnall Army Community Hospital at Fort Hood, Texas:

- *Every employee is to look for opportunities that would improve the result for the patient or the staff.*
- *Every patient is to be treated as though he or she were a member of the family.*
- *Decisions will be made at the lowest possible level.*
- *Problem solving will be marked by a high degree of staff and managerial communication, as well as by interdisciplinary input and collaboration whenever appropriate.*

Given principles such as these, if a staff nurse notices that patients are complaining about cold food on the unit, the nurse could form a team of nurses and food service aides to address the problem. If a housekeeper encounters a family who is trying to find some place to eat, the housekeeper can take the family directly to the cafeteria without having to ask permission from his or her supervisor or give elaborate instructions on how to navigate through the buildings. If a laboratory technician identifies blood specimen tubes that lack proper labelling in one unit, he or she could comfortably approach the nurse manager with the problem before it resulted in lost or repeated blood tests.

These examples point out the benefits of having guiding principles or value statements operationalized by each individual. They also suggest that quality-based strategic planning must make a difference in daily work at all levels of the organization, particularly the front lines where patients and quality-related problems are first encountered.

Approaches and Tools

Formulating the mission, vision, and guiding principles is not a linear process. Usually, the three are developed at the same time with much input from stakeholders of the organization.

The mission is usually developed by senior management and the board of directors. Quality concepts, particularly the meeting of customers' needs, must be interwoven into the mission statement. Hence, senior managers and the board should consider prior to drafting the mission statement *both* the market and the health needs of the community that the HCO serves.

The meetings to develop the mission statement are often facilitated by a consultant who assumes the roles of process expert and honest broker, ensuring that all viewpoints are considered. The agenda for meetings includes a framework which would answer the following questions:

- Who are we?
- What are we?
- Why do we exist?
- Who is our constituency? (or, Who are our customers and stakeholders?)

These questions also address the basic question, "Are we doing the right things?" which is the first of three critical questions for quality improvement submitted by The Hospital Research and Educational Trust's Quality Measurement and Management project (James, 1989). (The other two are: "Are we doing the right things right?" and "How can we be certain we do the right things right the first time, every time?")

Answering the specific question on the HCO's constituency is particularly important since it is the necessary precursor to the follow-up questions regarding the needs and expectations of stakeholders (the constituency) as will be discussed later in this chapter.

The formulation of the vision statement and guiding principles should be a highly collaborative endeavor among management, the physicians, and the workforce.

The most workable method first involves a draft by senior management or the steering council of the vision statement and guiding principles. This draft is then submitted to the rest of management, the medical staff, and the employees for their input.

Input can be obtained in a number of ways. The most common method involves sending a memo to the entire staff, with a draft of the vision and guiding principles as attachments. Responses are consolidated by either the planning office or the quality improvement office, and given to the steering council (SC) for consideration.

The preferable, but more time-consuming, alternative is the use of management and employee focus groups to obtain feedback on the vision and principles as was done at Optima Health in Manchester, New Hampshire. At Optima, the director of organization development facilitated meetings of five managerial and 28 employee groups, each of which were approximately three hours in length. After each group provided input on the vision and operating principles, the facilitator asked the group to identify how the vision and the principles could be applied in their particular work settings.

Asking for input is not done for the purpose of obtaining buy-in, but to acquire the insight from those closest to the customer and to make quality "real" for all employees. An example of this was demonstrated when a ward clerk said, "What quality means to me is that if my wife was admitted, she would be treated like she was the wife of the mayor."

Identification of Stakeholders

Stakeholders, or constituents, are those who have an interest in the organization and whose involvement the organization requires for success. They could be internal (employees, managers, physicians) or external (payers and patients). The Detroit Medical Center (DMC) identified 17 distinct stakeholder groups:

1. Patients.
2. Family.
3. Employees.
4. Trustees.
5. City Council.
6. Residents and fellows.
7. Medical students.
8. Managers.
9. Payers.

10. Attending physicians.

11. Referring physicians.

12. Suppliers and vendors.

13. Research institutions.

14. Volunteers.

15. Donors.

16. Foundations.

17. Accrediting agencies.

Stakeholder Needs and Expectations

After the organization's stakeholders are determined, the next step is to ascertain the needs and expectations of each. This is usually done in one of four ways.

The most common method is a survey or questionnaire sent to each group. The second and most time-consuming approach is a series of individual or focus group interviews. The third approach is having a representative from each group attend the HCO's strategic planning retreat. The fourth—and most preferred method—is a combination of all three, which would first consist of a survey of all stakeholder groups. This survey would be followed by individual interviews with key stakeholders (trustees, donors, and medical staff leaders), and focus group meetings with representatives of other groups. These individual and group meetings would allow further exploration of issues identified on the survey. Finally, representatives of all groups would be asked to present and discuss their needs and expectations at a planning retreat.

After the needs and expectations of all groups are identified, priorities are established and plans are put in place to meet or exceed these needs and expectations as will be described in the next chapter.

External Assessment

As part of the overall strategic planning process for the HCO, an extensive environmental assessment is made to identify threats to, and opportunities for, the organization. This external assessment, sometimes called the environmental scan, addresses such elements as the economy, political environment, market and competition, technology, and social or cultural variables.

In order to develop the quality plan, which will be part of the HCO's overall strategic plan, the following template is offered as a way to specifically consider external issues and questions which relate to the quality of care and the services provided:

External Assessment Template

1. **Health status.**
   a. What are the health needs of the community we serve?
   b. To what extent are we currently meeting those needs?

2. **Community resources.**
   a. What resources exist to address health needs?
   b. What are the gaps in providing care to the community?
   c. How can we collaborate with community agencies and other health care providers to meet these needs?

3. **Technology and knowledge.**
   a. What new or improved technology is available to enhance the quality of care we give to patients?
   b. What new administrative or clinical processes (e.g., clinical pathways, triage systems, patient-focused care, continuous quality improvement

tools) should be utilized to enhance the efficiency or access to care?

4. **Regulation, licensure, and accreditation.**
   a. What new regulatory, licensure, or accreditation requirements must be adopted?
   b. What accreditation requirements do we want to excel at as an organization, particularly to improve the quality of our services and our reputation in the community?

5. **Competition.**
   a. What is the reputation for service and quality of our competitors?
   b. What do we need to do to enhance our reputation for service and quality for the following key stakeholder groups: attending and referring physicians, our payers, and the community at large?

6. **Demographic and cultural variables.**
   a. What changes have occurred since our last assessment regarding the population we serve in terms of lifestyle and healthy behaviors?
   b. What are any new demands or expectations of the population we serve given any changes in demographics, culture, or attitudes?
   c. What demographic changes could affect our ability to obtain skilled workers?

7. **Healthcare financing.**
   a. What are the demands by the 3rd party payers regarding cost, price, and utilization?
   b. What will be the organization's response to these demands?
   c. How might the organization's response affect the quality of care?

d. What needs to be done to ensure that quality is not compromised by any cost-reduction initiatives taken by the organization?

Approaches and Tools

The external assessment for the quality plan is usually conducted by a task force consisting of staff from the quality and planning offices. The task force will take the results of the organization's larger environmental scan and supplement it with answers to questions from a template such as the one described above.

The task force integrates the results of the organizational environmental scan and the template along with any other feedback from other sources such as that from patient satisfaction studies and stakeholder assessments. The task force then recommends a prioritized list of external issues that affect the HCO to the HCO's strategic planning council. The strategic planning council then considers this assessment in conjunction with the internal assessment as discussed below.

Internal Assessment

An internal assessment provides information so that the organization can identify its capabilities to take advantage of opportunities and deal with threats from the external environment. In particular, an internal assessment will analyze the HCO's strengths (areas on which the organization can capitalize in order to reach quality goals) and its weaknesses (barriers to quality goals).

The assessment should be performed at least annually as part of the internal capability analyses conducted by the planning office. The assessment serves as an excellent means to: (1) establish a baseline or start point to begin quality efforts; (2) review the effectiveness of the organization's quality initiative; (3) prepare for a JCAHO survey; and (4) generate motivation in quality improvement or revitalize quality initiatives which may have been dormant due to other organizational priorities (e.g., restructuring, downsizing, merger activities).

Tools and Approaches

The following internal assessment template was developed and is presently being used by the author as a consultant. The template was designed based on a synthesis of Baldrige quality award criteria, the JCAHO performance improvement chapters, the Criteria for the President's Award for Quality and Productivity Improvement, and common assessment questions from the field of organizational development.

Internal Assessment Template

1. **Top management/leadership.**
   a. What is the current level of knowledge of quality improvement (QI)?
   b. Does top leadership lead the QI effort?
   c. What is the dominant leadership style and philosophy?
   d. Do department and service chiefs have ongoing QI efforts?

2. **Human resource development.**
   a. What is the current level of knowledge of QI?
   b. Are facilitators available and skilled?
   c. Are there incentives, rewards, and recognition for QI efforts?
   d. Are employees aware of the HCO's vision, mission, and values or guiding principles?

     e. Do employees know how the vision, mission, and values or guiding principles apply to them in their daily work?

3. **Medical staff.**
   a. What is the current level of knowledge in QI?
   b. Are QI approaches and tools being utilized to assess and improve clinical practice?
   c. What is the level of acceptance of QI on the part of the medical staff and their leadership?

4. **Employee empowerment and teamwork.**
   a. Do managers support employee empowerment and teamwork?
   b. Are employees empowered to take action to improve the quality of care or the services they provide?
   c. Are interdisciplinary teams utilized to address quality issues?
   d. Do employees use quality tools and approaches in their daily work?

5. **Structure and infrastructure.**
   a. Has QI been integrated with other quality functions such as risk management, utilization review, and infection control?
   b. Is there a mechanism or structure to oversee QI efforts?
   c. Are resources (e.g., FTEs, space, funding for training programs) for the QI effort adequate?
   d. Is there sufficient management information system (MIS) support for QI?
   e. Are QI efforts considered in light of other change efforts (e.g., downsizing, restructuring, organization development)?

f. What are the affects on QI from these other change efforts?

6. **Strategic quality planning.**
   a. Have long-term goals for quality been established?
   b. Is QI integrated with the strategic planning process?
   c. Has a QI or performance improvement (PI) model been adopted for the HCO?
   d. Have a clear mission, vision, and guiding principles that reflect quality concepts been established?

7. **Customer orientation.**
   a. Have all key internal and external customers been identified?
   b. Have customer needs and expectations been assessed?
   c. Are efforts taken to enhance customer satisfaction, particularly with respect to access, service, and communication with patients and their families?

8. **Measurement and analysis.**
   a. Have quality indicators been set?
   b. Is there a system for measuring, analyzing, and using the results of quality efforts?

9. **Results.**
   a. Have quality goals been met?
   b. What are the results of quality indicators?
   c. Do results show improvement from past years?
   d. What should be done differently if goals have not been achieved or if indicators point out that results have not met expectations?

The above template is usually used by external consultants who conduct one-on-one interviews with all senior managers and members of the quality and planing staffs. Group interviews are then held with a cross-section of middle managers and employees.

The results of the assessment are summarized by the consultants and submitted to the steering council (SC) for consideration. Often, the consultants present their findings as part of a SC retreat in which the issues and action items are discussed. After the SC retreat or meeting, members of top management brief the organization on the assessment and on the actions which will be taken.

If time for conducting interviews is limited, the above template can easily be converted to a survey with respondents submitting responses to each question. As another alternative, a shortened interview protocol is offered below. From experience, this abbreviated template has proved to be a highly effective way to obtain rich and robust information on the current status of QI, as well as ideas for future actions.

Internal Quality Assessment Template (Abbreviated)

1. How does QI work in the organization?
2. How does QI work in your department?
3. What is the current condition of the QI efforts?
4. What are barriers to the QI effort?
5. What are organizational strengths that we can count on to assist in future QI initiatives?
6. What needs to be done to make quality happen?
7. Are there any other comments you would like to make?

If the organization has the time and the desire to conduct an extensive assessment using standardized criteria, the management should consider using the guidelines of

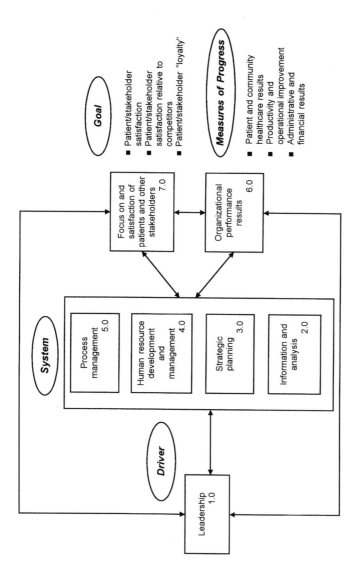

Figure 2.1 Healthcare Pilot Criteria Framework

Source: National Institute of Standards and Technology: 1995 Health Care Pilot Criteria, the Malcolm Baldrige National Quality Award (this material is in the public domain).

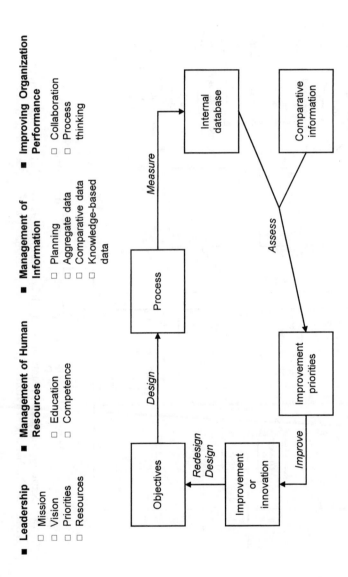

Figure 2.2 Critical Aspects of a Healthcare Organization's Internal Environment

Source: 1996 *Comprehensive Accreditation Manual for Hospitals*. Oakbrook Terrace, IL: Joint Commission on Accreditation of Healthcare Organizations (1996), p. 35. Reprinted with permission.

the Malcolm Baldrige National Quality Award. Figure 2.1 is a diagram which shows the basic elements, and the relationship among elements, of the Baldrige Award Pilot Criteria for Healthcare.

Anther excellent framework for the internal assessment is the JCAHO's Framework for Performance Improvement, which includes critical aspects of the organization's internal environment (see Figure 2.2).

Finally, there are short instruments (surveys) such as the TQM Inventory and the Climate and Readiness Survey from the Federal Quality Institute, which give a quick overview of the status of the QI effort, but lack in specificity and richness of data.

Summary/Roadmap of the Assessment Phase

Below is a summary or "roadmap" for the key tasks or activities during the first phase of quality-based strategic planning. As will be the case in all chapters, this roadmap represents the most generalizable or relevant approaches from the information and case examples discussed in the chapter. Additionally, the summary provides a "common thread" from the three case studies found in Chapter 7. Thus, this summary becomes a guide—a starting point for QBSP. A major caveat in its use is that it should be tailored to the organization's culture, structure, and resource constraints. Also, the user should realize that strategic planning is not necessarily a linear process. Often, the tasks within the same phase are accomplished simultaneously or combined as part of a larger activity.

A1. Establish a philosophy and structure for QBSP

   a. Have a broad view or philosophy of quality
      improvement which includes community health

status (e.g., incidence of disease), clinical quality (e.g., patient care outcomes), and service quality (e.g., admissions process, waiting times, responsiveness to third-party payers).

b. Establish a steering council (SC).
   1. Role: oversee the planning process, provide direction, allocate resources, approve the plan.
   2. Members: Senior management team and the directors of quality and planning.

c. Establish a resource group (RG).
   1. Role: conduct detailed analysis, coordinate QBSP initiatives, oversee training and facilitation, and monitor activities.
   2. Members: selected members of the planning, quality, and HR/training staffs; along with operational representatives.

d. Clarify roles.
   1. Quality improvement is everyone's job with every individual striving to improve quality in daily work.
   2. Department managers are owners of processes and systems, and thus ultimately accountable for process and systems outcomes.
   3. Executives and senior managers make strategic planning part of normal business since it is a standing agenda item at staff meetings.
   4. The SC and RG oversee, facilitate, and support the strategic planning process across the organization, particularly by providing guidance and coordinating efforts of departments and cross-functional teams.

A2. Review and/or establish statements of vision, mission, and guiding principles (see Appendix A for examples).

a. Establish statements based on input from across the organization.

b. To obtain specific comments from managers and the workforce, ask the following question when they are providing ideas or reviewing drafts: "What does the vision and each of the guiding principles mean to you?"

A3. Identify key customers and assess their needs and expectations.

a. Focus on five key customers for healthcare organizations are: patients, community, employees, physicians, and third-party payers.

b. Begin the assessment with focus groups of different customer groups to obtain in-depth knowledge, ideas for innovation, and firsthand feel of issues. Follow up with an extensive survey of all customers, particularly patients, employees, and physicians.

A4. Conduct an external assessment.

a. Examine seven key areas: health status, community resources, technology, regulation, competition, demographics, and healthcare financing.

b. Use a template to guide efforts (see External Assessment Template, page 24).

A5. Conduct an internal quality assessment.

a. Assess nine key areas: top management leadership, human resource development, medical staff, employee empowerment and teamwork, structure and infrastructure, strategic planning, customer orientation, measurement and analysis, and results.

b. Use a template such as the Internal Assessment Template (page 27), the abbreviated version (page 30), or the Malcolm Baldrige National Award Criteria.

CHAPTER 3

PLANNING

Planning takes the results of the internal and external assessments, including the stakeholder analyses, and considers these in light of the mission, vision, and guiding principles. The planning phase tends to be the most complicated since it must integrate numerous inputs and define themes or goals for improvement which are applicable across the organization. Then, once the goals are set, action plans are put into place to ensure that goals are met. Planning must fully consider all the nine critical elements for quality improvement, particularly empowerment—a recognition that the staff at all levels must understand, accept, and participate in the planning process.

Additionally, planning must ensure the alignment of department goals with those of the organization.

Steering Council (SC)

Planning is usually initiated, coordinated, and monitored by a steering council (SC) or a quality council (QC) which develops recommendations for the executive leadership (if different from the SC/QC). This group develops a planning process, ensuring that quality and strategic goals are integrated and that quality principles are followed. The group then facilitates and monitors the implementation of the plan throughout the organization.

Table 3.1 is an example of the role and functions of the Quality Council at Optima Health in Manchester, New Hampshire.

Table 3.1: Role and Principal Functions of the Quality Council, Optima Health

Basic Role: To facilitate change so that quality happens at Optima.

Principal Functions:

1. Establish quality philosophy, vision, and guiding principles.
2. Serve as advocates and champions for all quality efforts at Optima Health (OH).
3. Coordinate and oversee quality-based strategic planning.
   a. Assure that quality is planned into all activities.
   b. Maintain inventory of activities.
   c. Avoid duplication and link activities.
   d. Facilitate quality initiatives:
      (1) Assure that OH addresses strategic priorities.
      (2) Recommend priority/delay/"no go" on other initiatives requiring resources.
      (3) Sponsor specific quality/process improvement initiatives.
      (4) Charter process action teams and task forces.
      (5) Establish guidelines for submission of quality initiatives.
4. Secure and promote:
   a. XMT (executive management team) commitment/involvement.
   b. Medical staff involvement.
5. Support:
   a. Norms and values.
   b. Change management.
   c. Team building.
   d. Management development.
   e. Empowerment of managers and employees.
6. Train and educate:
   a. Establish a common language.
   b. Train in tools, skills, and techniques.
7. Provide facilitator resources.
8. Help secure other resources from within organizational structure and budget.

9. Remove barriers to quality improvement.

10. Reward and recognize individuals, teams, and departments for quality efforts.

11. Communicate:
    a. Needs for improvement.
    b. Activities.
    c. Ideas and methods, "brokering" of ideas and methods throughout the organization.
    d. Accomplishments (within the organization and externally).

12. Monitor and report progress:
    a. Of specific initiatives.
    b. Of the overall quality effort at OH.

13. Oversee and coordinate the work of:
    a. Quality management/utilization review steering committee.
    b. Continuum of Care Task Force.
    c. Patient Care Redesign Team.

There should be only one steering council for both strategic planning and quality improvement. The SC should consist of the senior leadership team (for an example, see Table 3.2).

Table 3.2: Steering Council Membership, Walter Reed Army Medical Center

— Director of Clinical Services (chair)
— Chief operating officer
— Chief, Department of Medicine
— Chief, Department of Surgery
— Chief, Department of Nursing
— Director of strategic planning and TQM

The SC/QC must be trained in quality improvement prior to undertaking the planning process. The following five topics are most critical:

1. TQM philosophy and concepts.

2. Applications and lessons learned from other health-care organizations.

3. The systems approach.

4. Strategic quality planning.

5. Ways to lead the quality effort in the organization.

To assist the SC/QC, a resource group is designated. This group provides assistance in such areas as formulating detailed plans (e.g., the roll-out plan); training; analyzing assessments of customer needs and expectations; and recommending quality indicators, improvement priorities, and process improvement teams. The roles and responsibilities of the Resource Group at Optima Health are listed in Appendix B.

Members of the working group reflect a cross-section of the organization. At Walter Reed Army Medical Center, members include the director of strategic planning and TQM, the assistant director for TQM, the TQM training coordinator, chief of nursing education, director of quality management, and two representatives from each of the nursing and medical staffs.

Overview of the Planning Process

An eight-step planning process is proposed:

1. Operationalizing the vision statement and values.

2. Review of the mission statement and strategic goals.

3. Analysis of internal, external, and stakeholder assessments.

4. Integration and identification of themes for improvement.

5. Establishment of quality goals.

6. Development of a roll-out plan.

7. Establishment of a budget.

8. Publication and dissemination of the plan.

Development of the above was based on experience and from a synthesis of five quality planning approaches as seen in Table 3.3.

Table 3.3: Five Quality Planning Approaches

Approach	Key Characteristics	Key Elements/Process
Juran Quality Planning	Quality plan separate but coordinated with the strategic plan.	"Roadmap" of identifying customers, assessing needs and expectations, and translating same into operations (identifying processes).
Hoshin planning	• Quality and strategic planning totally integrated. • Linkages of plans to department and individual goals.	Vision elements, break-through areas, annual objectives, catch-ball matrices, and reviews/audits.
Traditional strategic planning	• Top-down, driven by planning office. • Emphasis on financial, market, and competitor analyses.	Internal and external assessments, mission/vision statements, goals, strategies, action plans, and financial plans/budgets.
Baldrige award framework	• Criteria offered for quality improvement design and evaluation.	Leadership as the "driver"; system consists of process management, human resource development, strategic planning, and information and analysis; goals of customer satisfaction and organizational performance.
JCAHO's performance improvement framework/cycle	Focus on: relationship with external environ-ment, internal character-istics and functions, and method for assessing/improving functions and work processes.	Process design/redesign and performance measure-ment, assessment, and improvement.

As mentioned, all the approaches identified in Table 3.3 were considered in the development of the eight-step model for planning. A synthesis of these was made based on what has worked in health organizations—from the personal experience of the author and from reviews of case studies.

Although the eight steps are common to successful applications of strategic planning, the tools or techniques used in each step may vary depending on time availability and the culture of the organization.

The remaining discussion will focus on the tools and techniques that could be applied during each of the eight steps of the strategic planning process.

Step 1. Operationalizing the Vision Statement and Operating Values

The vision statement along with the statement of operating values are the best places from which to start the strategic planning process.

As identified in Chapter 2, the vision statement is the capstone for any strategy since it sets the future direction for the organization. Operating values provide constancy of purpose, giving all organizational members guidelines on how they will function as they move towards the vision and organizational goals.

Usually, when the organization undertakes QBSP, both the vision and operating values statements have been published. It is now necessary to "operationalize" the statements; that is, to make them more specific, applicable, practical, and concrete. It is also essential to identify the major tasks which must be completed to achieve the vision and guiding principles.

The first task requires clarification of all vision elements and operating values. Thus, the steering council must be sure it agrees to what is meant by such statements as "quality of service," "quality of working life," or "the provider of choice." This clarification is best obtained through asking a question from the perspective of the customer. The Sisters of Mercy Medical System (SMMS) uses an exercise with its senior management team that consists of writing a short article addressing the question: "If an article were written about SSMS five years from now, what would you want that article to say?" At SMMS, managers are divided into small groups to discuss this question. Then, responses are shared and reconciled in a open discussion.

Optima Health uses a variation of this approach by focusing more specifically on their quality improvement effort: "If an article were written about Optima's quality program five years from now, what would you want the headlines to say?"

At Optima, small groups of the Quality Council (QC) answered the question. Responses were shared with others on the QC. Additionally, this information was used later with other data to prioritize actions. The use of "headlines" was more appropriate for Optima due to time constraints and the ease of transferring the bullets ("headlines," as opposed to narrative) to other parts of the planning process during a quality planning retreat and later at QC meetings.

In order to begin to identify the major tasks and overall priorities for the organization, there is one basic question which must be asked: "What should be done to realize our vision?"

This question could be made more specific by asking, for example: "What must Good Samaritan Regional Health Center accomplish to become the premier healthcare provider in Southern Illinois?"

There are two other questions that generate much additional insight and information:

1. What would facilitate reaching our vision and operating values?

2. What things are getting in the way of achieving our vision and values?

Responses to all questions are then used by the steering council. The information will be combined with the results from the assessment phase and input from the other remaining planning steps as will be described below.

Step 2. Review of the Mission Statement and the Strategic Goals

Implications for quality improvement should next be identified from the mission statement and any strategic goals or initiatives which have already been published.

Unfortunately, in many organizations, quality goals are not included along with other strategic goals such as of increased market share and profitability. If quality goals are included, they usually tend to be broad statements about the organization's commitment to quality improvement. Thus, it is incumbent on the steering council to make quality happen. The council should consider three approaches:

1. The first (and most critical) approach is to make quality a specific strategic initiative or goal along with those dealing with market share, financial performance, managed care contracting, etc. It could well be that quality improvement could be a major force that enables the organization to reach other strategic goals.

2. The second approach begins with asking the question: "What are the implications for quality for each element in the mission statement and each strategic

initiative?" An excellent way to stimulate thinking around implications is to have guidelines or criteria. In conducting quality planning, Holy Cross Hospital (Silver Spring, Maryland), uses guidelines from the *Joint Commission on the Accreditation of Healthcare Organizations (JCAHO) 1996 Accreditation Manual*. In the manual, JCAHO identifies nine "Dimensions of Performance" (such as efficiency, appropriateness, and availability). At Holy Cross, critical processes are identified for each quality function (such as care of patients, management of human resources, and education). Teams are assigned to measure and improve each process. They must then consider each of the nine dimensions during their discussions using a checksheet.

3. The third (and least preferred) approach is taking each strategic goal and asking the question: "In reaching this goal, what do we need to do to ensure that quality of patient care is not adversely affected?" The reason this is the least preferred alternative is that it is defensive—*it does not plan for quality improvement*. It limits action only to ensuring that the current level of quality is not affected.

Step 3. Analysis of Internal, External, and Customer/Stakeholder Assessments

The results of the internal, external, and stakeholder assessments are provided to the steering council (SC) for analysis. The council can receive information in final or "raw" form (that is, with or without analysis and conclusions).

Usually, the data is provided in final form with statistical summaries and conclusions. The SC then reviews the information as a group and supports, changes, or makes additional conclusions based on their experience and insight or on new information about the external or internal environment. This is done by consensus from group discussions. If a number of implications are identified, these can be prioritized through multi-voting.

Sometimes the information is provided in raw form. In this case, the analysis is conducted by the planning/quality staff who usually identify a large number of strengths, weaknesses, opportunities, and threats to the organization. The council can best resolve this through the use of an affinity diagram in which issues can be categorized. The steps in constructing an affinity diagram are:

1. Individually brainstorming issues, writing down one issue per Post-it™ note.

2. Placing the Post-it™ notes on the wall.

3. Silently sorting the notes on the wall until categories emerge. Any member of the council can move the notes in a manner that they see best.

4. Labeling the categories by making a header that best describes the grouping of Post-it™ notes.

Finally, the prioritized categories or implications are used as input in the next step of the strategic planning process.

Step 4. Integration and Identification of Themes for Improvement

The steering council must now integrate multiple inputs from the steps described above. Without efficient integration, the council will suffer from information overload and will not be able to move on to prioritization and action planning.

The SC must particularly take the "big picture" view during this step. In doing so, themes must be identified from the following key earlier inputs:

1. Responses to the question: "What needs to be done to achieve our vision?"

2. Implications for quality improvement from the review of the mission statement and the strategic goals.

3. Conclusions from the analysis of the internal, external, and stakeholder assessments.

There are two basic methods to identify the major themes or areas for improvement. The first (and least efficient) way is to have SC members review all inputs individually. Each member identifies themes and priorities among the themes, and then shares his or her prioritized themes and priorities with the group. The group must now discuss and reconcile many different priorities (this process can be speeded up somewhat by multi-voting on the themes/priorities after all have been shared).

The second method uses the affinity diagram described previously. The inputs or results from the previous three steps are made into bullet items and placed on the Post-it™ notes on the wall of a conference room. The SC members then jointly review these inputs and develop headers to describe the theme.

At Optima, the themes ("high priority areas") were identified by affinity diagramming through answering the following question, which was adapted from Joel Barker in *Paradigms*:

> *"What is it that we can't do today, or aren't doing today that—if we could—would fundamentally change our business, our quality, or our service to key customer groups?"*

An example of an extremely efficient process for identifying themes and for planning, in general, is that from Walter

Reed Army Medical Center (WRAMC). At WRAMC, the facilitator simply projected the vision statement onto a screen and asked the SC to brainstorm the answer to the question: "What is getting in the way of our vision?"

In less than one hour, over 80 items were identified. During the next two hours, these items were grouped into seven major categories using the affinity diagram. The header of each of these categories became a strategic initiative and a task force was assigned to develop an action plan for each category/initiative.

Whatever approach is taken, the results of this step are usually finalized and expressed as:

- themes/areas for improvement; or
- strategic initiatives/imperatives; or
- key/critical success factors (KSFs or CSFs).

Thus, the establishment of any process action team or other quality initiatives is based upon, and aligned with, these key strategic or business initiatives.

Step 5. Establishment of Quality Goals

After the themes or areas for improvement are formulated, the organization must move on the establishment goals or objectives for each theme or area. The establishment of themes and goals gives the departments, cross-functional teams, and the workforce concrete targets on which to focus their efforts. Hence, the organization obtains the "biggest bang for the buck" by having alignment of goals at the team and individual employee levels.

There are three basic elements that should be addressed in setting quality goals:

1. Clear linkage with the themes, areas of improvement, key success factors (KSFs), or strategic imperatives.

2. Measurable end points.

3. Focus on results, rather than on activities.

Examples of goals include:

- Improve health status of the community by 10 percent as measured by epidemiology studies for alcoholism, teen pregnancy, and suicide.
- Reduce the average infection rate by 20 percent.
- Improve the overall satisfaction level as measured by the annual Gallup Survey by 15 percent.
- Meet all length-of-stay guidelines as negotiated with third-party payers.

The above examples focus on measurable end results, or outcomes. Too often, goals focus only on activities the ultimate purpose of which is unclear. Examples of this are:

- Establish four new health centers.
- Increase primary care physicians from 25 to 50.
- Institute clinical pathways for each medical procedure.

The above goals are inappropriate as stand-alone goals since they reflect only activities to achieve some larger end goal. Thus, the three examples above must be tied or changed to such goals as improved community health status, improved primary care, and clinical efficiency, respectively.

The setting of goals is usually accomplished by the SC in a discussion facilitated by the quality staff in a two- or three-hour meeting after the themes for improvement are identified. The goals developed by the SC are forwarded to the department chairs for their consideration. After this input is received, the SC reconsiders the goals and a final list is provided to the board of directors for approval.

Step 6. Development of a "Roll-Out Plan"

After goals have been established, a "roll-out plan" or a "quality roadmap" is needed to make quality happen in the organization. The goals and themes for improvement identified by the organization provide the backdrop for specific actions within the plan. An outline for a "roll-out" plan is offered below:

Roll-Out Plan Elements

1. *Themes for improvement, key success areas.*

2. *Quality goals.*

3. *Quality improvement concepts and models.*
    a. Overall approach to quality for the organization.
    b. Process improvement model for teams and individuals.

4. *Structure for quality improvement.*
    a. Composition and role of the steering council.
    b. Composition and role of the QI resource group.
    c. Role of the quality sub-committee of the board.
    d. Role of department managers.
    e. Linkages to the medical staff.
       i. Committees and meetings.
       ii. Role of department chairs.
    f. Linkages with other quality efforts and committees.
       i. Quality management (infection control, risk management, utilization management).
       ii. JCAHO accreditation survey.
       iii. Patient satisfaction (e.g., "voice of the customer").
       iv. Patient care redesign.
       v. Continuum of care.

5. *Process action teams.*
    a. Chartering of cross-functional teams by the SC.

  b. Chartering of department-specific teams.
  c. Linkages among teams, departments, and the quality
     structure.
  d. Reporting requirements.

6. *Training.*
  a. Executive and senior management training.
  b. Orientation training for all employees.
  c. Management "toolbox."
  d. Medical staff training.
  e. Facilitator training.
  f. Team training.

7. *Management information systems (MIS).*
  a. Development of a "quality management dashboard."
  b. MIS requirements to support measurement by
     teams, departments, etc.
  c. Role of MIS office.

8. *Human resource management.*
  a. Incentives for QI.
  b. Implications for the performance appraisal system.
  c. Team-building interventions to support QI efforts.
  d. Role of the VP, HR.
  e. Role of the director of organization development
     and training.

9. *Communication plan.*
  a. Information on the QI initiative provided to
     employees.
  b. Information to the board and the community.
  c. Establishment of progress reports to the board, med-
     ical staff, managers, and employees.

10. *Audit and review of quality initiatives.*
  a. Frequency of reviews.
  b. Use of Baldrige criteria.
  c. Role of the SC and the resource group.

The roll-out plan should be accompanied by a timetable that clearly outlines the sequence of its elements. The roll-out plan (and the timetable) should be submitted to all middle and senior managers for their review and input. The plan must be "their plan" as well, since quality is not a function limited to the QI office or a steering council.

When reviewing the plan, managers consider and provide feedback on its clarity, thoroughness, and any adverse impacts or arduous requirements on their units, such as the timing of quality initiatives conflicting with other anticipated events. This feedback is usually sent to the QI staff, which forwards issues to the next meeting of the SC.

Step 7. Establishment of a Budget

After the roll-out plan or quality road-map has been developed, its associated costs must be determined. Budget requirements must be approved by the steering council and sent for final approval as part of the normal budgeting process for the organization (customarily on an annual basis) or as a separate appropriation. The separate appropriation is usually needed if the budget request is submitted during the fiscal year for a mid-year start-up of the QI program or a new quality improvement initiative.

To ensure adequate funding, the budget should fully consider the following elements or line items:

- FTEs for the quality improvement and training functions (partial FTEs will be needed for in-house trainers).
- Consultant fees.
- Conference fees and travel to support professional development for the QI staff and SC committee members.

- Funds to support ongoing programs or special initiatives such as benchmarking studies and new quality measurement software, etc.
- Audio-visual and training materials (videos, student manuals, conference or training facility rentals).
- Funds to support team projects (e.g., pilot studies, start-ups of new processes).
- Funds to support recognition and rewards systems (e.g., "quality day," cash rewards).

Budget problems usually can be addressed at the SC meetings if the chief financial officer (CFO) is a member of the council. If not, the director of quality must usually submit the request through the normal budget process (and the ensuing debates), or make a personal appeal to the CFO, hopefully with the backing of the director's supervisor and other senior managers.

Step 8. Publication and Dissemination of the Plan

Once the budget is agreed to, the plan should be submitted to the CEO and senior leadership (if not represented on the SC) as well as the board.

After final approval, the strategic plan is published in one of three ways:

1. As a separate plan, usually called the "quality plan," "quality roll-out plan," or "quality roadmap."

2. As an appendix to the strategic plan.

3. As an integral part of the strategic plan in which quality initiatives are included alongside those involving cost reduction, patient access, managed care, etc.

However formatted or jointly published, the plan should he considered a working document. Thus, the document should be easily accessible and amenable for revision as necessary on the basis of new situations, opportunities, and customer needs and expectations.

Not everyone needs a copy of the strategic plan. However, every person in the organization must have some basic understanding of the purpose and nature of the plan. Additionally, parts of the plan or versions must be published in a form that is useful for different target groups. The distribution and communications strategies suggested for different groups are found in Table 3.4.

Table 3.4: Communications Strategy

Document/ Communications	Content	Target Group
Actual plan	Entire plan with time-table	All managers
Employee newsletter (announcing new QI plan/initiatives)	• Reasons for QI • QI model and structure • Key goals and initiatives • How to submit ideas for improvement	All employees
Letter to the medical staff	As above for employees	All physicians
News release	• Reaffirmation of commitment to QI and patient satisfaction • Key goals and initiatives	Community and third-party payers
Brochure/fact sheet	• QI model and structure • Key goals and initiatives • How to submit ideas for improvement	All managers, employees and physicians

The publication and distribution of the plan does not end the process of QBSP—the plan must still be implemented and its results evaluated, as will be discussed in the next two chapters.

Summary/Roadmap of the Planning Phase

P1. Establish a philosophy for planning, emphasizing the following elements.

a. Customers needs and expectations, particularly those of patients, the community (health status), employees, physicians, and third-party payers.

b. Analysis of customer needs and expectations, and market forces, to determine:

1. Strategic goals.

2. Focus of quality improvement (QI) projects.

c. Catch-ball—widespread involvement and participation in the planning process by all management levels and the medical staff.

d. Alignment of:

1. Mission, vision, guiding principles, and goals.

2. Strategic goals and QI projects.

3. Quality and financial planning.

4. Quality and cost-reduction initiatives (e.g., downsizing, restructuring, discharge planning and utilization review).

e. Cascading of goals throughout the organization.

f. Empowerment and accountability—giving managers and the workforce the authority and responsibility to develop and carry out goals consistent with the strategic objectives of the organization.

g. The organization as a system:
  1. Focus on strategic interests of the overall organization.
  2. Integrate plans across the organization (avoiding suboptimization of specific functional areas or product lines).
  3. Consider impacts of any goals or action plans on all parts of the organization.

P2. Operationalize the vision statement and values.

a. At a strategic planning retreat ask:
  1. "If an article were to be written about our facility five years from now, what would you want that article to say?" This question will help people in the organization focus on (or add to) key areas in the vision statement.
  2. "What does our organization need to do to realize our vision and operating values?"
  3. "What is getting in the way of realizing our vision and values?"

b. During planning sessions at the department level, ask:
  1. "What does the vision and values statement mean to our department?"
  2. "What do we need to do, given the vision and values?"

P3. Review the mission statement.

a. Ensure that quality improvement is made an explicit part of the mission statement. Consider JCAHO's nine "Dimensions of Performance" as mission statement elements:
  1. Efficacy.
  2. Appropriateness.

3. Availability.
4. Timeliness.
5. Effectiveness.
6. Continuity of care.
7. Safety.
8. Efficiency.
9. Respect and caring.

b. Identify the implications for quality improvement for each element of the mission statement at a steering council meeting, then solicit additional input from all members of the management team.

P4. Analyze internal, external, and customer/stakeholder assessments.

a. Information from all assessments is summarized by the resource group (RG) for consideration by the steering council (SC).

b. The SC categorizes and prioritizes issues through the use of affinity diagramming and multi-voting.

P5. Identify areas of improvement and key success factors (KSFs) or strategic imperatives (SIs).

a. The SC considers the following inputs:
   1. Results from operationalization of the vision and values (Step P2).
   2. Results from review of the mission statement (Step P3).
   3. Internal, external, and customer/stakeholder assessments (Step P4).

b. The SC identifies and names KSFs and SIs via "themes for improvement" (seven or fewer, to maintain focus and optimize resources):

1. Each member looks for themes for improvement across all inputs.

2. Each member presents his or her recommended themes for improvement, and the SC discusses commonalities and differences.

3. The SC prioritizes themes by asking the key question, "Of these, what are critical to our success?" Should the group have difficulty in coming to consensus on themes, the QI tools of affinity diagramming and multi-voting are recommended.

P6. Establish quality goals.

a. Quality goals are set for each KSF or SI.

b. Criteria for quality goals:

1. Directly relate to and measure a critical aspect of each KSF or SI.

2. Directly relate to and measure critical areas of concern for each customer group (e.g., patients, physicians, employees).

3. Are measurable.

4. Focus on results rather than on activities.

c. The goals are then reviewed by the departments for their input and comment ("catch-ball").

P7. Determine quality projects.

a. Ideas for quality projects are generated by:

1. The SC and RG as they review all assessment data and identify themes for improvement (P5b).

2. Department managers as they review the KSFs, themes for improvement, and the quality goals as part of the "catch-ball" process.

3. Individuals by giving input via surveys, focus groups, and the suggestion program.

b. Evaluate and prioritize quality ideas and projects:

1. Ideas are collected and initially studied for merit by the RG.

2. The SC reviews recommendations for projects from the RG.

3. The SC prioritizes projects using group consensus (or multi-voting) based on the degree to which the projects support one or more of the KSFs/SIs.

c. Quality projects are forwarded to either departments (e.g., reducing ER waiting times), committees (e.g., infection control, safety), or cross- functional teams or task forces to address issues that affect many departments or services (e.g., admitting and discharge processes, patient flow through intensive care units). (Detailed information on quality projects is provided in the roll-out plan.)

P8. Develop a roll-out or implementation plan for QI.

a. Purpose: To provide a single-source document to guide the QI effort.

b. Key elements of the plan (a detailed outline of a plan from one organization is found in "Roll-Out Plan Elements" on page 50) are:

1. Organizational philosophy of quality.

2. Structure for quality improvement.

3. Quality goals.

4. QI projects.

5. Process action teams.

6. Departmental responsibilities.

    7. The individual's role.

    8. Measures and measurement strategy.

    9. Information systems support.

    10. Training programs.

    11. Use of facilitators.

    12. Rewards and recognition.

    13. HR, organizational development, and team-building.

    14. Communications and marketing plan.

    15. Evaluation of QI initiatives.

    16. Resource requirements to support the plan.

c. Other parts of the plan include time frames and responsibilities for completion of each element of the plan.

d. Process: The plan is developed by the RG, reviewed by department managers, and submitted to the SC for final approval.

P9. Establish a budget.

a. Resource requirements (the last part of the roll-out plan) are carefully reviewed by the SC, of which the CFO is a member.

b. Separate appropriations may be needed to support the following resource-intensive areas:

    1. Training.

    2. Quality projects and benchmarking studies.

    3. Rewards system.

P10. Publish and market the plan.

a. Target key groups: employees, department managers, and physicians.

b. Create communications and marketing strategies (see Table 3.4).

CHAPTER 4

IMPLEMENTATION

*"Any dammed fool can write a plan. It's the
execution that gets you all screwed up."*

— Lt. General James F. Hollingsworth

"We strategize beautifully, we implement pathetically."

— Anonymous

Implementation is the most important aspect of QBSP. For
the strategic plan to work, four critical areas must be
addressed:

1. **Leadership.** The most crucial functions during
   implementation are leadership behaviors and the
   role senior management plays in establishing organizational culture, communication, rewards, support structures, and policies.

2. **Departments.** Department managers must align the
   strategic plan and goals with those of the department. Additionally, they must obtain commitment
   to the goals and quality initiatives.

3. **Individuals.** The workforce must not only be committed but have skills to carry out quality and

customer service improvements and be equipped to adapt to change.

4. **Cross-functional teams.** Since most issues in health organizations cross departmental lines, cross-functional or interdisciplinary teams should be formed to address key systems issues such as the admission, discharge, and patient flow processes.

Leadership

The speed and the degree to which plans are implemented are mostly dependent on leadership. Existing attitudes, values, vested interests, and the longstanding way of doing things cause considerable inertia and pose strong resistance to change.

Leaders must be change agents. Thompson and Strickland provide the best summary of necessary leader behaviors. He states that the strategy-implementer's "action agenda" involves:

> *Communicating the case for change to others, building consensus for how to proceed, installing strong allies in positions where they can push implementation along in key organizational units, urging and empowering subordinates to get the process moving, establishing measures of progress and deadlines, recognizing and rewarding those who achieve implementation milestones, reallocating resources, and personally presiding over the strategic change process.*

A recent article in *Harvard Business Review* suggests that a major reason why TQM (and business process reeningeering) fails to reap full benefits is that it often does not address management processes—"the ways senior managers make, communicate, implement, monitor, and adjust decisions, and measure and compensate performance" (Beyond, 1995, p. 80). This implies that leaders must be committed to TQM; establish an appropriate rewards and incentive system; and communicate, model, and follow up on desired behaviors.

Other authorities have described other leadership approaches which have been shown to be effective in the implementation of change, particularly with respect to organizational culture:

- Peter Senge speaks to the need for a shared vision in his book, *The Fifth Discipline*. This is achieved through involvement, communication, and discussions about the vision and values for the organization.

- Tom Peters and Nancy Austin in their book, *A Passion for Excellence*, emphasize the value of "MBWA"—"management by wandering around," which allows the manager to provide direct, consistent, and reinforcing communication on changes to subordinate managers and employees.

- Edgar Schein, in *Organizational Culture and Leadership*, maintains that organization change requires cultural change and that culture is strongly influenced by symbols, stories, myths, rituals, and the style of the leader or founder.

This writer has taken these ideas and merged them with Lewin's (1951) longstanding model of change. This model consists of three phases:

1. Unfreezing the current state, condition, or behaviors.

2. Shifting to a moving state.

3. Refreezing or locking-in new behaviors in the new state or condition.

Incorporating each phase, a model for a step-by-step change strategy is given below. This model has been used by this author in the implementation of numerous change efforts, ranging from reorganization to the deployment of computer systems on nursing units.

Implementation/Change Strategy Template

Phase 1: Unfreezing.

a. Assess the readiness for change, including any reasons why individuals or groups are resistant.

b. Communicate the advantages of the change, directing communication toward the existing values and beliefs.

c. Allow individuals to go through the "grieving process" by having them express their sorrow, fears, and concerns about leaving the past. (One manager had a "funeral" by having employees participate in the burial of the old policy manual.)

Phase 2: Moving.

a. Involve staff in devising solutions to issues and concerns about the transition. (The maxim "people will support what they help create" is operant here.)

b. Set objectives and milestones to give the staff foreseeable and reachable goals.

c. Empower the staff (now that goals have been established) to decide how to reach the goals.

d. Align norms and values. (For example, avoid announcing that the staff is empowered while still requiring a sign-off by senior managers before any change is permitted.)

e. Align goals and rewards. (For example, do not set a goal of improving quality of information to patients and families, yet still reward the patient representatives and phone operators for the number of calls handled.)

f. Implement the change.

g. "Walk the talk" and practice MBWA—"management by wandering around"—by providing continuous, consistent, and supportive communication.

h. Assess the impact of the change on your staff and other parts of the organization, making revisions to the implementation plans as appropriate.

Phase 3: Refreezing.

a. Have fellow employees and managers (through user groups, staff meetings, etc.) and informal leaders encourage, reinforce, and model the new desired behaviors.

b. Reward and recognize staff for demonstrating the desired behaviors and carrying out the change, avoiding the "folly of rewarding A, while hoping for B" (Kerr, 1995). Hence, if teamwork is valued, managers should reward team (as opposed to individual) accomplishments.

c. Celebrate success and establish rituals (such as annual parties on the date on which key goals were reached).

d. Publish procedures that institutionalize the new way in which things are done.

e. Monitor, evaluate, and continuously improve.

The list below is a summary of the key, specific action ("The Big 10") that a leader should take during the implementation phase:

1. Receive training in quality improvement, then become a trainer.

2. Be visible, "walk the talk," and serve as a role model for quality.

3. Empower subordinate managers and employees to innovate and identify improvement opportunities.

4. Align goals, values, and rewards.

5. Recognize and reward desired behaviors.

6. Follow up on the roll-out plan.

7. Include QI as a specific agenda item at all staff meetings. (This will keep QI on the front burner and make QI a part of daily operations.)

8. Monitor key processes.

9. Play catch-ball—involve your staff in coordinating initiatives across the organization.

10. Have a customer focus, constantly seeking ways to exceed needs and expectations.

Departments

For purposes of this book, departments include all organizational subdivisions such as services, programs, and product lines.

Departments are often quite large and complex. For example, the department of nursing usually has over 50 percent of the FTEs of a hospital and a number of specialty units including the operating rooms, intensive care units, and labor and delivery rooms. A community health program could have over 200 staff positions. A department of medicine in a medical center has usually 12 subspecialities including cardiology, gastroenterology, endocrinology, and hematology/oncology.

Hence, given their size and the fact that departments, services, or programs deliver the work of the organization, it is imperative that quality improvement be made an integral part on their ongoing operations. Experience has shown that the following elements are crucial in departmental quality improvement efforts:

- Quality improvement coordinator.

- Quality improvement plan.

- Mechanisms to improve quality, particularly cross-functional teams.

- Training for the entire organization.

Quality Improvement (QI) Coordinator

Ideally, the QI coordinator would also be the department head. However, in large departments such as nursing or environmental services, a separate coordinator is usually appointed.

The person has the functions of coordinating all planning, training, quality meetings, and quality team activities within the department. The quality coordinator reports directly to the department head but also has a "dotted line" relationship with the organization's QI director. Communication between QI coordinators and the QI director centers around:

- Information on organization-wide quality initiatives and plans.

- Reports of quality initiatives and plans within the department.

- Department issues that need organizational attention.

- Coordination of the work of departmental and organizational project teams.

- Discussion of training needs for the department.

Quality Improvement Plan

Each department should have a quality improvement plan which is aligned with that of the organization. The plan would define the department's quality goals, quality indicators, and the key actions to reach quality goals. Additionally, departmental plans will usually include a section on training which will outline how and when managers and employees will be trained in quality improvement. An excellent example of departmental planning and deployment has been submitted by Fontana, Butcher, and O'Brien (1994) based on their experience at The George Washington University (GWU) Hospital.

Another example is at Walter Reed where this writer (in the capacity as director of strategic planning and TQM) facilitated planning meetings for all clinical departments. The process used for departmental planning is outlined below:

Departmental Planning, Walter Reed Army Medical Center

Step 1. Participation of the department director in the organization's strategic planning retreat, in which organizational goals and strategic initiatives were determined.

Step 2. Training of department and service directors in the planning process at Walter Reed and the basic concepts of quality improvement (QI), the use of groups in QI and planning, managed care, and cost reduction. The training was conducted by the director of strategic planning/TQM and the director of managed care.

Step 3. Development of a draft departmental plan at a series of meetings attended by the department director, subordinate service chiefs, and the director of strategic planning/TQM. These meetings (usually two four-hour meetings) consisted of the following (in addition to individual preparation by department director and service managers and documentation by department/service secretaries):

a. A joint briefing by the director of strategic planning/TQM and the department director to the service managers on organizational goals and initiatives.

b. Discussion of implications of organizational goals and initiatives on the department and the services within the department.

c. Development of goals and plans in support of each organizational initiative.

d. Identification of issues to be forwarded to the steering council regarding any additional resource requirements or adverse impacts of organizational initiatives.

e. Presentation by all service managers on goals and initiatives for their service and ideas for department wide goals/initiatives. (These are listed by the facilitator on flip charts and posted throughout the room.)

f. Clarification and discussion of ideas for department goals, including service goals that have a major impact on the department and organization, particularly those which require additional financing or space.

g. Achievement of consensus on departmental goals through group discussion or by multi-voting.

Step 4: Presentation of the department's goals at a retreat attended by the steering council and all department directors. At this meeting, each department director defends his or her plan and the other department directors provide comments and then anonymously evaluate each department goal or initiative on a one-to-five scale.

Step 5: Based on the input from Step 4, the steering council approves, denies, or returns the department plan for modification.

Mechanisms to Improve Quality, Including Teams

Each department should determine by what means quality issues and opportunities are identified and resolved. A most practical and effective way is to make quality improvement an agenda item at each staff meeting. This way, QI always remains on the front burner.

A more elaborate, but time consuming, method is for the department to have its own steering council with meetings separate from the usual staff meetings. Departmental steering councils are most appropriate for large departments since their staff meetings tend to have many staff in attendance and lengthy agendas. Thus, to give QI the attention it needs, a separate meeting or council is suggested for large departments.

Another critical means to address quality issues and opportunities is for the department to charter its own project teams. These intra-departmental teams deal with issues primarily affecting one department, whereas cross-functional teams deal with issues that affect a number of departments. The problem, of course, becomes how to coordinate the activities of all the departmental and cross-functional teams. As mentioned previously, this coordination is achieved through meetings in which the QI director and all departmental QI coordinators are present.

Training

Training for QI in departments consists of three programs: management development, team training, and individual training, which will be discussed in the next section.

Department managers should be provided a tool-kit—a set of skills that enhance their ability to plan and improve quality.

Unfortunately, management development is often uncoordinated, fragmented, and scattered throughout the organization. This is because management training is often separately conducted by the human resources office, the QI office, and by the large departments, particularly nursing.

For maximum effectiveness, one comprehensive management development program should be designed in which key management skills, including those involving QI, are taught. An example of a management "toolbox" for one organization is provided below.

Management Development Program

1. Review of managerial roles.
   a. Translating corporate goals to operational goals.
   b. Improving quality and reducing costs.
   c. Addressing employee issues.
2. Management skills.
   a. Planning and problem-solving.
   b. Team building and conflict management.
   c. Change management, overcoming resistance to change.
   d. The learning organization and systems approach.
3. Leadership skills
   a. Employee motivation.
   b. Dealing with fears and lack of risk-taking.

    c. Management-by-wandering around (MBWA).

    d. Empowerment and reinforcement of Covey's "Seven Habits."

    e. Communication and listening skills.

4. Cost and efficiency.

    a. Management engineering, workflow analysis.

    b. Profiling, pathways, etc. to enhance clinical efficiency.

    c. Cost of poor quality.

    d. Addressing the cost versus quality issue.

5. Running effective meetings.

    a. Meeting design (setting the agenda, ground rules).

    b. Meeting management tools.

    c. Facilitation skills.

    d. Running "town-hall" meetings.

6. Quality improvement.

    a. QI concepts.

    b. Process improvement.

    c. QI tools (e.g., nominal group technique, flow-charting, cause-effect diagramming).

    d. Establishing a culture and environment for quality.

7. Customer service.

    a. Improving customer service and access.

    b. Using Gallup data and other customer input.

    c. Supporting and developing the "front lines."

8. Applications and open discussion.

    a. Case studies/examples from other healthcare organizations.

    b. Open discussion on issues identified by participants.

Individuals

An organization and department should strive for all employees to be committed to and have the skills to support quality improvement and customer service. Commitment to quality is achieved through leadership as discussed previously. The skills for quality improvement and customer service are achieved largely through training, supplemented by role modelling, counselling, and reinforcement by managers in the department.

The writer's experience and a review of the literature have identified the following topics in common with successful QI training programs for employees:

1. The QI philosophy, approach, and initiatives in the organization and the department.

2. The individual's role in improving quality.

3. The importance of teams and teamwork, and of viewing fellow employees as customers.

4. Techniques to assess and improve one's own work and effectiveness.

5. Means to submit quality ideas through the chain of command and the QI structure of the organization.

6. Communicatng and dealing effectively with patients, the patient's family, and fellow employees.

An example of a program for employees who work on the frontlines of care (such as clinic receptionists and ward clerks) is found in Table 4.1. The program, which was delivered by this writer and a colleague to over 500 individuals in a variety of healthcare organizations, emphasized customer service, communication, and self-empowerment skills and included a session on diversity issues in dealing with customers.

Table 4.1: Customer Service—Quality from the Grass Roots (Course Objectives & Outline of Topics)

1. To motivate employees on the importance of customer and staff relations:
   - Review/primer on TQM philosophy and concepts
   - Who is the customer?
   - Why is customer service so important?
   - The price for dissatisfied customers
   - The ten myths of customer service
   - The employee's role as an internal customer and supplier of services
   - The employee's role in creating a positive image
   - The employee's role as a first-line problem-solver
   - The employee's role as a team member
   - The ten most common mistakes made by employees in customer relations (e.g., rudeness, not caring, appearance)

2. To understand how the employee's personality affects customer relations:
   - Administration of the Myers-Briggs Type Indicator (MBTI)
   - Feedback and discussion of each personality type
   - Development of a personal strategy for change

3. To develop empowerment skills on the part of each employee:
   - Problem-solving
   - Communication techniques
   - Conflict management
   - Time management
   - Personal organization
   - Use of TQM on a daily basis

4. To develop specific customer relations skills:
   - Answering phones and greeting customers
   - Using phrases, voice techniques, and body language to build rapport
   - Handling inquiries and complaints
   - Dealing with anger
   - Managing appointments and schedules
   - Managing multiple demands from customers, your boss, and other staff

- Maintaining a favorable and friendly work environment
- Obtaining customer feedback
- Pinpointing customer concerns, then quickly addressing these
- Interacting with the public relations office
- Role plays on the above

5. To acquire sensitivity to diversity and cross-cultural issues:
   - Valuing age, gender, ethnic, and cultural differences
   - Building on the strengths of diversity/differences
   - Diversity/cross-cultural exercise

Cross-Functional Teams

Most quality problems and opportunities for improvement are not confined to one department. Accordingly, individuals representing different departments must be brought together to address major systems issues within the organization. The formal structuring of such a group is called a cross-functional team. These teams confront large, complex, and crucial process issues such as the flow of patients through the health system.

Use of teams requires considerable attention to formation, membership, organizational linkages, group dynamics, training, and resources. A cross-functional team should not be formed unless basic criteria are met. Forming teams without clear purpose and need will waste valuable organization time and cause the QI program to lose credibility. Experience has shown that the following four criteria, phrased in questions, are essential:

1. Does the team support a strategic or quality initiative?

2. Does the team have potential for improving patient care, access, and/or customer satisfaction?

3. Would more than one department be affected?

4. Is there an issue that is not being addressed by another group or department?

Membership in a cross-functional team should be based on who can provide critical input on the problem and its resolution. The team leader is the one who has the primary responsibility for the process or issue being examined.

Cross-functional teams, like departmental teams, must receive training in QI concepts, processes, methods, and tools. In addition, teams should devote time to team-building, since members have probably not worked together previously. Experience has shown that team-building should be conducted with respect to issues of goals, roles, relationships, and group norms. If these issues are not systematically addressed through the team-building process, the team flounders miserably for the first two or three meetings.

The team must also be clear on reporting and coordinating relationships. To assist the team in this regard, the steering council usually appoints a liaison to ensure that the team:

1. Carries out its charter or mission.

2. Moves efficiently toward goals set by the SC.

3. Submits timely reports.

4. Coordinates efforts with other teams, departments, committees, and task forces in order to share ideas and prevent suboptimization of any one process.

5. Has sufficient training and resources to carry out its mission.

It has been found that the liaisons have been key in tying efforts of teams together, particularly in ensuring that quality goals set down in the implementation plan are met.

Summary/Roadmap of the Implementation Phase

I1. *Establish a philosophy for quality implementation, emphasizing the following principles.*

    a. Quality improvement is everyone's job.

    b. Leaders/managers are owners of organizational processes and systems.

    c. There is coordination of quality initiatives across the organization ("horizontal catch-ball").

    d. Practice management-by-wandering-around (MBWA).

    e. Implementation is the hard part of quality-based strategic planning; thus considerable effort must be put in to initiating actions and follow-through on plans.

I2. *Executives' role.*

    a. Receive training, then take part in QI training as a trainer.

    b. Be visible, "walk the talk," and serve as a role model for quality.

    c. Empower subordinate managers and employees to innovate and to identify QI opportunities.

    d. Align goals, values, and rewards.

    e. Recognize and reward desired behaviors.

    f. Follow up on the roll-out plan.

    g. Include QI as a specific agenda item at all staff meetings (this will keep QI on the front burner and make QI a part of daily operations).

    h. Monitor key processes—you are the owner.

    i. Play catch-ball, involving your staff and coordinating initiatives across the organization.

    j. Have a customer focus, constantly seeking ways to exceed needs and expectations.

I3. Department managers' role.

    a. Same as above.

    b. Further develop key management skills (see the Management Development Program on page 71).

    c. Conduct departmental planning, aligning goals with those of the organization (see example of a departmental planning process on page 68).

I4. Role of each individual.

    a. Seek out ways to improve quality in daily work.

    b. Forward ideas to management, the RG, or through the suggestion program.

    c. Participate in process action teams and quality improvement projects whenever possible.

    d. Attend training (see Table 4.1 for an example of training program geared to the front-line workforce).

I5. Role of the cross-functional teams.

    a. Carry out the charter defined by the SC.

    b. Receive training as a team on the quality improvement process, problem-solving tools, and team-building.

    c. Ensure that measures of success are defined.

    d. Document and report results.

    e. Obtain input from supervisors and fellow workers

prior to team meetings and keep them informed of team progress.

16. Role of the resource group.

a. Assist cross-functional teams with start-up, including group membership, training, team-building, and facilitation.

b. Monitor activities of the cross-functional teams.

c. Coordinate efforts, serving as a liaison among teams and departments.

d. Design and conduct training programs (usually accomplished by members who have expertise in training design and delivery, such as those in areas of employee, managerial, or organizational development).

e. Receive and initially evaluate all ideas for quality improvement projects.

f. Assist department managers in their quality efforts.

17. Role of the steering council.

a. Charter quality improvement teams.

b. Evaluate and approve recommendations for new quality projects.

c. Provide for and adjust resources as necessary to carry out QI projects.

CHAPTER 5

EVALUATION AND CONTINUOUS QUALITY IMPROVEMENT

"Quality is a race without a finish line."

— David Kearns, former CEO, Xerox
(Schmidt & Finnigan, 1992)

Organizations cannot stand still and rest on their laurels. The implementation of plans must be followed by an evaluation of what is working or not working and why. Additionally, the organization must document what has been learned and use those lessons in future quality improvement efforts. Finally, the health organization must innovate and relentlessly pursue the improvement of quality, employing the philosophy and concepts of continuous quality improvement (CQI).

Sustaining things that work, improving existing processes and systems, and designing innovative new services will ensure that the organization stays ahead of the competition by meeting the changing customer or market needs. The organization and its departments, cross-functional teams, and individual employees must all continuously evaluate, sustain, improve, and innovate as discussed below.

Organizational Evaluation

What to Measure

Measures for each quality goal are established during the planning phase. The degree of attainment of each goal should be carefully tracked and monitored by the steering council. However, there are other measures of importance which need to be tracked. Among these are items of interest to third-party payers, government, accrediting agencies, and professional associations.

The government at the state or local level might require HCOs to report on such items as programs that monitor access to emergent care or primary care for the indigent. Additionally, the government might encourage quality initiatives such as the New Hampshire Patient-Centered Care Project in which hospitals follow patients to determine the impact of medical care in their daily living and functioning (Morrissey, 1996, pp. 64-65).

The Joint Commission on Accreditation of Healthcare Organizations (JCAHO) has provided new impetus to system measures which reflect processes and functions that cross departments and involve a wide variety of disciplines. For example, Holy Cross Hospital has established measures for each of the functional chapters of JCAHO's Comprehensive Accreditation Manual for Hospitals (CAMH). Thus, using the manual as a guide, measures have been established for such critical functions as the assessment and care of patients, patient and family education, and the continuum of care.

The JCAHO has also provided an excellent framework and guidelines for measurement which incorporate the JCAHO model for performance improvement as seen in Figure 5.1.

A number of other accrediting agencies, professional societies, and managed care plans have devised what are commonly called "report cards," which contain results of surveys of items of concern to consumers and payers. Among the most notable are the Group Health Association of America's Consumer Satisfaction Survey and the National Committee on Quality Assurance's Health Plan Employer Data and Information Set (HEDIS). In a recent study sponsored by the US Department of Health and Human Services, the following were deemed most important for monitoring with respect to the delivery of care:

1. Technical quality (skills of the provider).

2. Provider communication and interaction.

3. Accessibility of care (includes waiting times).

4. Continuity of care.

5. Clinical outcomes (the degree to which medical care had the desired effect) (Research Triangle Institute, 1995).

Finally, the organization should evaluate the effectiveness of any new design, process, or service such as a short stay unit, ambulatory surgery center, or wellness center. When these are designed, a determination should be made concerning what would constitute a quality operation or program. The characteristics to be evaluated would include: degree of use, acceptance and satisfaction by staff and patients, and comparisons to the previous (or any similar) method.

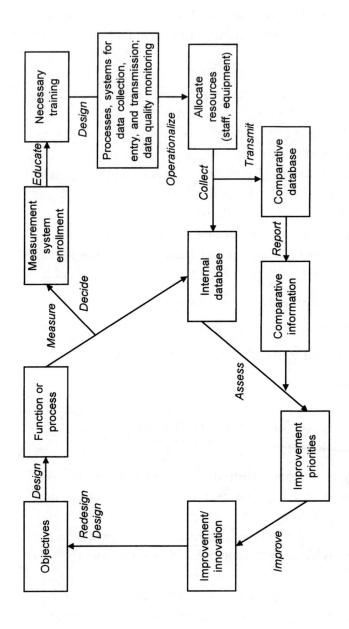

Figure 5.1 The Indicator Measurement System and the Cycle for Improving Performance

Source: *1996 Comprehensive Accreditation Manual for Hospitals.* Oakbrook Terrace, IL: Joint Commission on Accreditation of Healthcare Organizations (1996), p. 38. Reprinted with permission.

Analysis of Measurement Data

All these measures provide a wealth of information for the organization. However, they can be burdensome to analyze unless the results are analyzed and presented in a useful form. Collecting and analyzing the data is usually the responsibility of the resource group, which presents summary information to the steering council.

In analyzing the data, the group uses MIS tools such as spreadsheets, and QI tools such as trend analysis, run charts, and control charts. An excellent source for the analysis of data, particularly the application of statistical process control, is the book *Measuring Quality Improvement in Healthcare* (Carey and Lloyd, 1995).

Additionally, the resource group must consider the combined impact of trends associated with multiple measures as well as the differences among measures. Examples of these include patient satisfaction differences on different units and the joint impact or implication of low satisfaction rates on multiple units. The results of this analysis are then presented to the SC for consideration.

The Dashboard or Scorecard

Critical data on vital measures should be frequently updated and continually presented in a manner similar to displays of data on a car's dashboard. The car's dashboard usually includes vital information such as speed, remaining fuel, and engine temperature. Likewise, the organization should have vital pieces of data readily available for senior leadership. Kaplan and Norton (1996) maintain that organizations need a "balanced scorecard" that has performance measures in the areas of finance, customers, internal business processes, and learning and growth. Given this framework, such measures for an HCO might include weekly or monthly run charts on:

- Third-party collection rate and supply costs (finance).
- Overall patient satisfaction (customers).
- Wait times in the emergency room and the ambulatory care center (internal business process).
- Employee satisfaction levels and attendance at training sessions (learning and growth).

Steering Council Review and Action

In performing its evaluation function, the SC usually considers: the "dashboard" and other result measures; reports from the cross-functional teams and the departments; status of the roll-out plan implementation; and the cost-effectiveness of all quality improvement efforts.

1. Analysis of "Dashboard" Results

The SC evaluates changes in measures, comparing these to benchmarks, if appropriate, and ascertains the reasons for measures failing to meet expectations. The reasons are determined by the collective judgment of the SC members, using such tools as forcefield analysis or the cause-effect diagram. The identification of root causes is crucial, since it pinpoints the corrective action to be carried out by management.

2. Reports from the Cross-Functional Teams and the Departments

The SC should receive monthly summaries of the status of the teams it charters. For example, at Walter Reed, monthly meeting summaries consisted of the following elements:

1. List of attendees.
2. Review/corrections to previous minutes.
3. Discussion.
4. Conclusions.
5. Follow-up actions.

6. Next meeting (date, time, and location).

7. Status of progress towards team goals.

8. Issues requiring attention of the steering council.

Additionally, the SC should receive briefings from the teams. In both cases the SC evaluates how efficiently the teams move towards their goals, eliminates obstacles in their way, and redirects the teams' efforts on the basis of new information or circumstances.

With respect to the departments, the SC should monitor (on a quarterly basis) the status of departmental plans. This will again ensure that the departments are moving towards the goals they have set, thus supporting the departments in overcoming any barriers to success.

3. Status of the Implementation/Roll-Out Plan

The organization should conduct quarterly in-progress reviews or milestone reviews on the implementation of the roll-out plan.

At Walter Reed, the steering council paid particular attention to the status of the organization's seven strategic initiatives:

1. Patient needs and expectations.

2. Work climate.

3. Systems integration.

4. Organizational enhancement.

5. Graduate medical integration.

6. Military–medical readiness.

7. New or alternative mechanisms for care.

In the experience of this writer, the reviews served to continue the momentum in the above-listed areas. Additionally, the reviews identified actions that required change in organizational systems to support the strategic initiatives. For example, the steering council directed changes in management information systems (quality indicators), management development (additional training in team building and customer service), and funding (allocations for pilot studies).

4. Overall Cost-Effectiveness

In conducting an overall evaluation of the strategic quality planning effort, a very basic question should be asked—"Is TQM worth the effort?" The steering council and all affected stakeholders want a return on their investment—to recoup the costs of training and consultant fees, as well as the time spent in quality planning, process action teams, etc.

A thorough review of literature by Bigelow and Arndt (1996) revealed no empirical evidence that TQM works or does not work since there were no common and comprehensive measures of quality and no studies that rigorously looked at cost-benefits (some looked at costs and not benefits, others focused on benefits and not the costs). However, anecdotal articles suggested that TQM is beneficial in terms of customer satisfaction, profitability, productivity, service quality, and employee satisfaction.

A way of addressing the lack of evidence of cost-effectiveness is through the concept, "Cost of Quality" (COQ). COQ is defined as any costs incurred due to either bad quality or efforts to ensure good quality. It is measured by the sum of four components:

1. Prevention (quality planning, process improvement/ redesign, training);

2. Appraisal (inspections);

3. Internal failure (rework, bottlenecks, downtime, etc.); and

4. External failure (complaints, lawsuits). (Gupta and Campbell, 1995, pp. 43-49).

In evaluating effectiveness, reviewers should examine where expenditures on quality improvement are being made. Clearly, the most cost-effective category is prevention. Prevention lowers the costs of appraisal by reducing the need for inspections and lowers the probability of external failure—and the resultant high costs of lawsuits and poor image associated with adverse medical outcomes.

Bohan and Horvey (1991) submit that most organizations could save ten dollars for internal failures and up to one hundred dollars for external failures for every one dollar invested in prevention. Unfortunately, most of the quality expenditures (between 50 percent to 90 percent, according to Juran, 1989) are on the categories with the lowest payback—internal and external failures.

Another approach to examining cost-benefits in healthcare is offered by Castañeda-Méndez (1996) in a practice called "value-based cost management." It provides an excellent framework for evaluating costs with respect to structures, processes, and outcomes.

Evaluation within Departments

The evaluation function for departments can take a variety of forms. Probably the most effective method, which is also the simplest and yet most overlooked, is the staff meeting. Staff meetings tend to focus on dissemination of information (usually bad news), an immediate crisis, or urgent problems. These meetings should be expanded to include a brief review of the following three areas:

1. How effectively the department is meeting its quality goals and performing relative to indicators.

2. Feedback received from customers (particularly patients, physicians, and other departments).

3. Opportunities to improve quality.

When the above-listed items are discussed as part of the staff meeting, quality improvement moves from the back to the front burner and becomes an integral part of the day-to-day business of the department.

In addition to regular staff meetings, the department should consider an audit of service quality on a semi-annual basis. As part of the audit, the department discusses opportunities for improvement, as well as such obstacles to service quality as time delays, frustrations with system inefficiencies, and confusion on the part of patients and then families regarding hospital procedures, physical layout, etc.

Finally, to tie all quality efforts, including evaluation, together, the department should designate a quality coordinator. The coordinator would carry out the following functions:

- Monitor and report on department indicators and the status of quality goals.
- Evaluate the functioning and progress of department-specific quality teams.
- Coordinate quality efforts with other departments and quality teams throughout the organization.

Evaluation by Cross-Functional Teams

"The work of healthcare is done through teams of people."

(Ulschak and SwowAntle, 1995)

Teams should continually evaluate two aspects of their performance: (1) their effectiveness, which concerns the degree to which the team is meeting its charter and time frames as defined by the SC and their own goals and (2) how well they function as a group.

This review is best accomplished by the team at the end of each meeting by simply asking two questions:

1. Are we meeting our goals?

2. How could we work more effectively as a team? In actual meeting situations, the questions most likely to be asked are: "How did it go today?" or "Do we need to do anything differently?"

To assist the team in evaluating its progress, a liaison is usually appointed to the team from the resource group. As found in Appendix B, below are the key evaluation roles performed by the liaison from the resource group at Optima Health:

1. Reviewing the charter with the team.

2. Monitoring progress, identifying problems to be reported to the QC (Quality Council).

3. Observing team meetings and evaluating the team facilitator.

4. Insuring the team is ready for presentations to the QC.

5. Reviewing monthly and quarterly reports of team progress.

A more formal review should be done monthly by the liaison in reviewing the monthly progress report to the SC. If the liaison or the team identifies problems in group dynamics or team functioning, a team-building assessment should be conducted. One of the most useful tools for this assessment is the survey of group effectiveness developed by Schein (1988). This has been successfully used by the author for both team-building and analysis of group problems. The eight elements of the survey (Schein, 1988, pp. 57-58) are:

1. Goals.
2. Participation.
3. Feelings.
4. Diagnosis of group problems.
5. Leadership.
6. Decisions.
7. Trust.
8. Creativity and growth.

Teams should also elicit feedback from their customers, while conducting pilot studies, and after full implementation of changes. Inova Health of Springfield, Virginia has developed a management information system which continually allows the organization, particularly its teams and departments, to know how well they are fulfilling expectations via monthly surveys of customers.

Evaluation of Individuals

On a day-to-day basis, all staff—particularly those on the front lines of care—must make quality happen. Their combined efforts and commitment to quality will result in a true quality organization. A breakdown in any of the "thousands of moments of truth" (Carlzon, 1987) during the one-on-one encounters with customers throughout the day could cause the customer to lose faith in the entire system. Consider the customer's reaction to any of the following incidents:

- Surliness on part of the parking attendant.
- Confusing directions from the admitting personnel.

- Use of jargon and lack of full explanations by providers.
- Ward clerks who fail to forward messages to family members.
- Phone calls which are not returned by administrative or clinical offices.
- Retaking blood samples because the originals were mislabeled or lost.

It is recognized that the behaviors described above could be partially explained by stress and overwork, poor systems and failed leadership. However, individuals cannot absolve themselves from responsibility for their actions. Hence, systems must be in place to identify and correct individual performance problems. In addition, evaluations should be conducted to assess the degree to which individuals are participating in QI efforts and using QI methods in their daily work.

The following checklist has been developed in order to evaluate the effectiveness of QI efforts with respect to individual employees. This evaluation is typically done by the resource group on behalf of the steering council.

Checklist of Evaluative Actions for Employees

1. Based on a review of performance evaluations and surveys of managers, has job performance changed since attending QI training?
2. Based on customer feedback, what are the trends with respect to complaints and compliments about employees regarding customer service from patients, families, physicians, and other departments?
3. Based on surveys of the individuals themselves:
   a. Do they feel more competent to address QI issues and opportunities?

    b. What QI tools were used by the individual in daily work?

    c. What skills need to be enhanced?

    d. How have they operationalized the organization's vision and quality goals in their daily work?

4. To assess the extent of empowerment, what are:

    a. The trends in the numbers of ideas submitted by individuals at different levels of the organization?

    b. The trends with respect to lower-level employees serving on cross-functional teams?

5. To what degree do supervisors nurture the QI skills that employees learn through role modeling, providing peer mentors, and emphasizing customer service at meetings and in performance evaluations?

6. To what degree are individuals committed to their own growth and development as measured by use of library material on QI and by participation in self-study programs offered by the QI, HR, or other offices?

The Most Important Evaluative Questions

Whether evaluation is conducted on an organizational, departmental, cross-functional team, or individual level, two questions should always be asked:

1. What is getting in the way of patient care or customer service?

2. What can we do about it?

Keeping these questions on the front burner is critical to creating an environment and culture of continuous quality improvement, thus ensuring an ongoing competitive advantage for the organization.

Transfer of Learning

The lessons learned from the answers to the above-listed questions and from carrying out QI projects and activities must be captured so that they can be shared and appropriately applied throughout the organization.

This capturing and transferring of QI information is one of the crucial roles of the resource group. This group obtains information regarding their monitoring function through reports and from the collection of lessons learned via liaisons to cross-functional teams and from QI coordinators and/or managers in every department. This information is usually passed on through newsletters, electronic mail, team and department meetings, and individuals as they complete one project and share their knowledge with others.

Clearly, documenting and disseminating information on QI activities, results, and lessons learned are major steps in becoming a true learning organization.

Summary/Roadmap of the Evaluation and CQI Phase

E1. Maintain a philosophy for evaluation and CQI.

    a. Quality is a "race without a finish line."

    b. Innovation and the relentless pursuit of quality allow the organization to stay ahead of the competition.

E2. Establish a measurement "dashboard."

    a. Show measures that reflect the critical aspects of each strategic imperative, quality goal, and customer group.

b. Show measures of critical organizational processes or functions (e.g., wait times, accounts receivables, patient education).

c. Show measures that determine progress towards objectives for process action teams.

d. Show quality indicators for each department.

E3. The SC regularly reviews the following:

a. Results of the "dashboard" and other outcome indicators.

b. Implementation of the roll-out plan, particularly the status of strategic initiatives.

c. Progress of the process action teams and departmental plans.

d. Individuals' level of competence and commitment to quality improvement (see checklist on page 93).

e. Overall cost-effectiveness of quality improvement efforts, considering a cost-of-quality (COQ) initiative.

CHAPTER 6

CURRENT ISSUES AND IMPLICATIONS

Three major issues dominate the literature regarding the healthcare industry today: managed care, downsizing (restructuring), and mergers and acquisitions. Each can seriously affect healthcare quality. Below is a brief discussion of these issues and their implications for planning.

Managed Care

Issues

Recent articles have suggested that medical outcomes and patient satisfaction may be adversely affected by managed care's emphasis on cost. Ware et al. (1996) found that the elderly and chronically ill poor patients had worse outcomes in HMOs than in fee-for-service systems. Anders (1996) submits that managed care companies select hospitals and physicians primarily on the basis of cost. He states that for those with serious heart conditions, "managed care companies have repeatedly opted for what is cheap at the expense of what is best." According to Magnusson and Hammonds (1996), major employers, such as Xerox and GTE, have become concerned that the push towards lower costs went too far and that their employees' health may be affected. Additionally, employers, workers, and other consumers express difficulty in making decisions on the quality of the health plans they are offered, due to limited information for making comparisons.

Implications

Quality improvement (particularly measurement) is now a growing counter-movement to the previous juggernaut of cost reduction. There are several implications for managed care plans, employers, and hospitals, which are presented below.

Healthcare plans should carefully monitor the health outcome of vulnerable subgroups, particularly the elderly and the poor, and develop a balanced scorecard which explicitly includes both cost and quality indicators for all patient groups. Additionally, health plans should participate in external comparison databases, seek accreditation by outside agencies such as the National Committee on Quality Assurance (NCQA), publish specific results of all reviews, and affiliate with others who share a commitment to quality improvement.

Employers and consumers should continue to demand data on clinical outcomes and service factors (waiting times, percentage of denials, etc.). Magnusson and Hammonds (1996) cite the following examples of the renewed interest and steps taken with respect to quality by major companies.

- GTE uses health outcome experts to visit each of the company's 125 managed-care contractors in order to provide a "report card" so that employees can compare their quality.
- Marriott has established criteria for the selection of HMOs with quality criteria counting for 70 percent of the total selection score.

- Pepsico demands that HMOs participate in continuous quality improvement activities.

- US Air audits care of their employees and compares this against nationwide data.

- Xerox requires HMOs to provide comparative outcome data. Employees then use this information to select a plan. The workers will receive a bonus if they chose a plan that meets quality criteria.

Hospitals, in their efforts to reduce costs and become more competitive to managed care plans, should explore ways in which cost could be reduced while maintaining or even improving quality. Among those having the most promise are clinical pathways (incorporating practice guidelines), case management, and utilization review studies in which cost and quality are fully considered. For example, St. Mary's Hospital in Richmond, Virginia chartered a team called the "Cost Busters," consisting of both clinical and administrative staff. The team's mission was to identify ways of reducing costs without affecting quality or laying off staff. At Optima Health, Manchester, New Hampshire, the institution is expanding the role of the Ethics Committee to include the ethical considerations of cost reduction options. Dartmouth Hitchcock Medical Center in Lebanon, New Hampshire, has made a commitment to form partnerships only with organizations (including managed care plans) that share their commitment to TQM.

Downsizing and Restructuring

Issues

The major concerns regarding downsizing or restructuring are the effects on quality and morale. Specifically, it has been argued that the replacement of RNs by unlicensed personnel (e.g., nursing aides or patient care technicians) could adversely affect the quality of care (Kunen, 1996, Murullo, 1995). With regard to downsizing, Ruback (1995, pp. 23-28) submits that the remaining employees ("the survivors") have feelings of anger, depression, fear, distrust, and increased anxiety about their jobs and the organization. As a result, they tend not to take risks, share information with co-workers, or work openly in teams, but lose commitment to the organization—a scenario which is counter to maintaining or improving quality.

Implications

As mentioned previously, hospitals should establish mechanisms in which quality planning becomes part of any cost reduction initiatives. Thus, "maintaining or improving quality" should be a criterion in decision making at all management and staff levels. Additionally, hospitals which have replaced RNs with technicians and nursing aides should consider the establishment of quality indicators specific for each nursing unit to insure that proper standards of care will continue to be met.

In order to address the human cost of downsizing, particularly worker anxiety and new working relationships, organizations should consider such interventions as team-building and increased information and communication from management. Employee forums (discussion groups) and increased leadership training for front-line supervisors are also useful. With regard to restructuring/downsizing that results in fewer layers or numbers of managers, consideration should be given to development programs which focus on stress management, change management, team-building, and worker empowerment.

Mergers and Acquisitions (M&A)

Lessons from the Banking Industry

M&A activity clearly dominates the healthcare industry today as a strategy for survival in a highly competitive marketplace. However, the banking industry has had a much longer experience with mergers and acquisitions—and has identified a number of issues and implications which must be considered. For example, during merger activity, Hayes (1996) submits that "quality initiatives often end up on the shelf. There is no time for quality meetings, problem solving, or continuous improvement; everyone is simply trying to survive." Bruno (1995) found that merger activity often results in poor employee morale, personality and cultural conflicts, and challenges to maintaining high-quality services.

In order to manage this change, Farmer (1996) states that a new statement of mission, vision, goals, and guiding beliefs should be developed and clearly articulated. Also, managers need to support this statement with actions, new polices or programs, and reward systems.

Moreover, it has been found that an effective TQM process can facilitate a smooth transition from two companies to one. Says Hayes (1996), "The basic pillars of a successful corporate quality management process— interdepartmental communication, cross-functional teamwork, and detailed process analysis—are the very ingredients needed to make a merger successful."

In a panel discussion on strategies during times of M&A, banking leaders shared the need for clearly focused strategy on targeted market segments, shared vision and culture, outstanding customer service, and employee development to carry out new strategy, vision, and culture. In particular, the panel emphasized interventions with respect to human resources. Says Richard Kovacevick, CEO of Norwest Corporation, "Attract, develop, retain, and motivate diverse, talented people." John McCoy, CEO of BankOne states: "The company's competency-based programs produce a pool of qualified individuals for each critical position in the company and serve as a vehicle to evolve and reinforce our culture, values, and strategy across geographic lines." ("Strategize, Survive, and Succeed," 1994).

Farmer (1996) strongly encourages assessment of employee perceptions and views on what they think is important. He uses an example of one merger in which the assessment revealed that employees of both companies had placed an emphasis on customer service, although a number of differences were perceived in management style and practices. Thus, customer service became a focal (and effective) point for managing the transition and bringing together differences in management approaches.

Issues in Healthcare

Increasingly, healthcare organizations are merging with each other to form integrated health systems that will facilitate a continuum of care, reduce excess capacity, and provide a broad range of services to benefit consumers and to appeal to third-party payers. Dravone and Shaley (1995) state that if benefits are maximized, integrated systems can result in better access, reduction of "customer search costs," and standardized approaches to quality. Taylor et al. (1995) suggest that mergers can provide more resources to improve quality and reduce costs through such means as the sharing of best practices and use of combined databases on population groups and medical outcomes. Unfortunately, the benefits of mergers do not come without growing pains.

Taylor et al. point to the problem of a conflict of cultures. They give the example of United Healthcare and MetraHealth where the former "has a strong focus on quality and tends to be higher priced compared to MetraHealth." They go on to note that "rarely does a new culture arise; the dominant culture of the acquirer often prevails." The risk, of course, is that the acquirer will have a cost orientation which will dominate over quality improvement and service.

Also Taylor et al. (1995) and Bergman (1994) state that merging organizations tend to focus on the short-term and administrative concerns or tasks of the merger. As a result, quality initiatives get delayed and leaders often lose sight of customer needs. Says Roger Chaufournier, former assistant dean at John Hopkins University School of Medicine, "What they [the leaders] don't understand is that a TQM framework can help develop the management system needed to make the integration work" (Bergman, 1994).

Implications

TQM concepts can greatly facilitate the transition to an integrated organization. Conrad and Shortell (1996) state that during periods of mergers and rapid growth, organizations require a culture that allows for innovation, risk-taking, learning from mistakes, staff involvement, and team building. Thus, TQM's emphasis on customer focus, group problem solving, and empowerment are extremely valuable in creating a favorable environment or culture for change. Additionally, the TQM tools of flowcharting, forcefield analysis, and activity network diagramming greatly support efforts in the integration of key processes (e.g., admissions, billing, etc.) of the merging organizations.

The efficacy of TQM's concepts and tools in merger activity was documented by Bergman (1994) in the case of the joint venture between Columbia/HCA based in Louisville, Kentucky and Southwest Texas Methodist Healthcare System in San Antonio, Texas. In this case, the two organizations held a retreat with 45 attendees representing different levels in both organizations. A facilitator divided the participants into groups. Through the use of the TQM techniques of Hoshin planning and small-group meeting management, the participants came to a consensus on the new system's direction, customer demands, market trends, and organizational strengths, weaknesses, opportunities, and threats (Bergman, 1994).

Case Example—Optima Health

As will be discussed in greater detail in Chapter 7, Optima Health was formed as a result of the merger of the parent companies of two Manchester, New Hampshire hospitals: Elliot Hospital (Elliot) and Catholic Medical Center (CMC). In addition to the two hospitals, Optima Health encompasses other entities, including home healthcare, a regional laboratory, and the New England Heart Institute.

When the merger was approved, Optima set up a merger management office to facilitate the integration of the hospital and all functions. Four major integration activities occurred with respect to strategic quality planning.

The first was the development of a new vision, mission, and values statement (see Appendix A). This statement served as an excellent focal point for all stakeholders, particularly employees, physicians, and the community at large. Additionally, the process by which the statement was developed engendered a collaborative environment among all entities at Optima. The process consisted of three phases: (1) input from all employees of all entities via small group meetings; (2) drafting of a statement using this input by a team representing all entities; and (3) review and approval of the draft statement by upper management and the Board of Directors.

The second initiative was the development of a common model, language, and plan for quality improvement. A quality improvement model was developed by a task force which examined all existing models being used by Optima entities, as well as other models from a literature review. The task force, which had representation from all entities, adopted a unifying model based on the clinical model of assessment, planning, implementation, evaluation. The task force later became the nucleus of the Resource Group (RG). The RG then further facilitated integration through the design of common curricula for all QI education courses. In the process of designing these courses, definitions and, hence, a common language emerged for quality improvement. Finally, the RG developed an implementation plan for all quality improvement activities at Optima.

The third initiative was the integration of all quality functions (TQM, risk management, safety, case management, utilization management, etc.) under one umbrella. All of these quality functions were previously separate within both hospitals. Thus, this was an opportunity finally to bring together all quality-related functions (and two quality departments), thereby maximizing the resources of all entities. Again, this reorganization was achieved through a task force consisting of representatives of all quality functions in both facilities.

The fourth intervention is the ongoing benchmarking of processes from the two hospitals. Thus, processes such as scheduling, admitting, and discharging patients are being reviewed at both sites. The best practices of each are being incorporated into designs for new processes which will be standardized for both hospitals.

Although not directly related to strategic quality planning, other interventions were taken at Optima, including employee town-hall meetings, adoption of new medical staff bylaws, and employee surveys regarding issues of the merger and job satisfaction.

CHAPTER 7

CASE EXAMPLES

Optima Health, Inc.—A Case Example in Initiating and Sequencing Quality Planning Activities

Background

Optima Health was formed in February 1994 as a result of the merger of the parent companies of two local Manchester, New Hampshire hospitals: the Elliot Hospital and Catholic Medical Center. The merger, unique in that it brought together the only two hospitals in the city, received strong community support and an extensive review and ultimate approval from the US Department of Justice's Anti-Trust Division and the New Hampshire Attorney General's Office. The merger received support because it would better channel efforts towards community needs and result in cost savings by elimination of duplicative services.

Optima Health operates a healthcare system across the continuum of care. In addition to the hospitals, Optima Health consists of: home health services, a regional laboratory, New England Heart Institute, physician practices, a retirement community, adult daycare, and an ambulatory surgery center.

Vision, Mission, and Values Statement

Prior to the start of strategic planning, Optima undertook an extensive process to develop its vision, mission, and values which resulted in the statement found in Appendix A. This statement served as an excellent focal point for strategic planning efforts and established the basis for a collaborative environment at Optima.

The process for developing the vision, mission, and values was facilitated by the human resources/organization development offices. It consisted of three phases:

1. Input was sought from all employees via a series of 24 small group meetings over a four-month period with over 950 employees (approximately one-fourth of the workforce) from all levels and all departments and member organizations. Each group identified:

   a. A mission statement.

   b. A vision letter (letter written to a friend describing the organization in the year 2004).

   c. A value story (anecdote that shows how a particular value was demonstrated in the organization).

2. Drafting of a vision, mission, and values statement by a team consisting of 18 individuals from a cross-section of the organization. This team received the output from the 24 small groups and synthesized this information into a draft statement.

3. Review and approval of the draft statement by the executive management team, senior management team, and the board of directors.

A similar process is now being used to develop a vision, mission, and values statement for each department and member organizations. Thus, Optima's vision, mission, and values statement serves as the overarching guide for alignment of all statements across the organization.

Quality-Based Strategic Planning

In mid 1995, Optima's executive management team (EMT) determined that the quality efforts needed to be revitalized. In the previous year, merger activities and other immediate operational demands had taken precedence over quality improvement activities at the strategic or corporate level. Additionally, the EMT and the quality, planning, and human resource staffs strongly felt that a unified approach to quality planning and improvement was needed, particularly since different models and strategies were used at the organizations that merged to become Optima. Finally, the EMT decided that quality-based strategic planning and renewed efforts in quality improvement would simply be the right thing to do, and would result in a strategic advantage for the organization.

Below is a description of the sequence of events and major interventions undertaken during the period August 1995 through July 1996. Specific time frames are provided to assist the reader in planning and conducting a similar intervention. Additionally, the Optima example will show the models, tools, and other information critical to the start-up there.

Step 1: Assessment

An assessment was made over a three-day period in September 1995. Interviews were conducted with all members of the EMT and managing directors of large departments or services. Additionally, focus groups were formed which consisted of trustees, the quality staff of the two hospitals, human resource/organization development (HR/OD) staff, administrative assistants, and chairs of the medical departments.

The three objectives of the assessment were to define the current approaches to quality improvement at Optima, obtain input on the direction and strategies for QI in the future, and identify barriers to the planning and implementation of a new QI effort. The results of the assessment would be used in the strategic planning process and in the identification of training needs.

In August, an extensive interview protocol for the assessment was written (see Figure 7.1). However, when the interviews were actually conducted, the most meaningful and critical findings were derived from the following three questions:

1. What is going well in QI at Optima or your department?

2. What isn't going so well in QI?

3. What should be done differently in the future?

Step 2: Feedback

Feedback on the assessment results was provided in three meetings. The first was with the CEO and president; the second was with the entire EMT, and the third was with managing directors. In all three situations, the same feedback was provided and discussed. The key questions these meetings addressed were: "What are the themes from the assessment findings," and "What are the implications for action?" Responses were then later used by the consultant, the quality council, and a quality improvement task force in developing improvement plans or topics for QI training.

Figure 7.1: Interview Questions: Quality Assessment

Objective 1: Understanding, ideas, opinions

a. How do you see the quality improvement effort working at Optima Health (or your organization)?

b. How do you see the quality improvement effort working in your department, activity, of area of responsibility?

c. How does quality improvement fit in with strategic planning at Optima Health (or your organization)?

d. Given the past and what you hear, where is quality improvement going at Optima Health (or your organization)?

Objective 2: Barriers, strengths, and weaknesses

a. What is working about quality improvement that shouldn't be changed (e.g., strengths of the program)?

b. What needs to be changed or done differently (e.g., weaknesses of, barriers to, and gaps in the program)?

c. Has quality been affected in any way as a result of the merger, downsizing, cost-cutting, etc.?

Objective 3: Recommendations

a. Generally, where should the quality improvement effort be going?

b. Should the quality improvement function be structured or implemented differently?

c. Should the quality improvement function be integrated or linked with other functions (e.g., strategic planning, management development, marketing)?

d. What time frames seem reasonable for quality improvement implementation and the changes you have identified?

e. Specifically, what opportunities do you see for quality improvement given the issues at Optima or within you area of responsibility?

f. What are your thoughts on how Optima can balance among the issues of cost reduction, quality, and access/patient satisfaction?

Step 3: Formation of the Quality Council and Initial Meetings

The list of members of the QC is found below. Selection was based on what departments or individuals (a) had the power to effect major systems change or allocate resources to the project; (b) could provide input and effect change from major administrative, clinical, and community services; and (c) whose support of TQM efforts was crucial (such as marketing and information services).

Membership of the Optima Quality Council

- Chief executive officer.
- President.
- VP, chief financial officer.
- VP, chief operating officer.
- VP, medical staff affairs.
- VP, TQM and non-acute services.
- VP, human resources.
- VP, marketing/system services.
- VP, ambulatory/community services.
- Managing director, chief information officer.
- Chief nurse executive.
- Physician representatives (4).

After members of the QC were identified, the consultant met with each member in mid February 1996 to solicit ideas regarding the council's purpose and roles, and to identify agenda items for the initial meetings.

The first meeting of the QC was on February 22, 1996. The following issues were addressed:

(1) Determination of role and functions (see Table 3.1).
(2) Clarification of organizational linkages (see Figure 7.2).
(3) Establishment of ground rules (see Table 7.1).

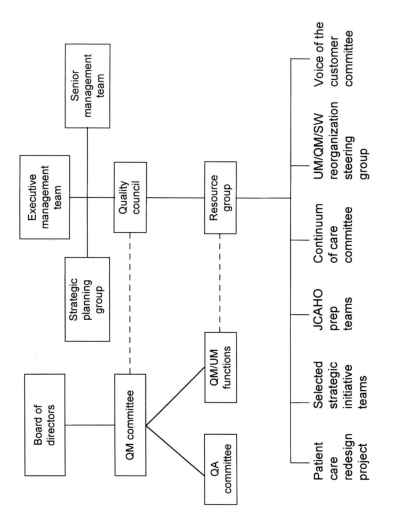

Figure 7.2 Quality Council Relationships

Table 7.1: Ground Rules for QC Meetings

1. Participate
2. Start and stop on time
3. Confront issues
4. Agree to disagree
5. Seek clarification
6. Focus
7. Do what is right, not what is easy
8. Support decisions
9. Maintain confidentiality ("What is said here stays here")
10. "Maintain an open chair" (available to CEO or other person as requested by the QC)

The second meeting, on March 25, 1996, produced the following:

1. The decision to move forward with the development of an electronic bulletin board for team reporting and sharing of QI activities, results, and lessons learned across the organization.
2. The finalization of topics for QI training.
3. The approval to develop training programs for managers, facilitators, teams, medical staff leaders, and those working on the front lines of care and service.

Step 4: Training of the Quality Council

A list of potential topics was drafted by the consultant and the VP, TQM & acute services, then presented to the QC at their first meeting for review and decision. The result was the curriculum in Table 7.2 which was presented as part of a one-day retreat on April 10, 1996. Training occurred in the morning and quality planning in the afternoon.

Training was conducted in an interactive fashion with the consultant presenting concepts and approaches, followed by questions and comments by members of the QC. Items that could not be immediately answered or resolved were placed in a "parking lot" for consideration during the afternoon or later planning sessions.

Table 7.2: Topics for Training of the Quality Council (QC)

TQM philosophy and concepts

TQM applications and case study

Quality-based strategic planning

The systems approach

Clinical vs. managerial orientations (implications for TQM)

Structure for TQM

Criteria for teams or task forces

Chartering teams

Coordination of TQM across departments

Monitoring teams and other TQM activities

Training and development (programs for managers, workers, teams, facilitators, etc.)

Leadership (creating a quality culture: "walking the talk," empowerment, use of champions, rewards, and reinforcement of training)

Step 5: Strategic Quality Planning

The planning process began on the afternoon of April 10, 1996, immediately following the training described above. The process consisted of a four-part sequence, each of which had a central question.

Part 1: Establishment of a vision for quality improvement at Optima by using small groups to answer the question: "If an article were written about Optima's quality program five years from now, what would you want the headlines to say?"

Part 2: Identification of "gaps" from the quality assessment by asking the entire group: "Based on the assessment, what action is required?"

Part 3: Identification of needs and expectations of customers by asking small groups: "What are the needs, expectations, and issues with respect to our five key customer groups of patients, the community, employees, physicians, and third-party payers?"

Part 4: Identification of high priority areas by the QC using the affinity diagram after each individual recorded his/her responses on Post-it™ notes to the question: "Given the results of the previous exercises and considering our mission, vision, and values, what is it that we can't do today, or aren't doing today, which, if we could, would fundamentally change our business, quality, or service to our key customer groups?"

The above process resulted in numerous action items for follow-up. Sub-groups of the QC met between council meetings in May and June 1996 to develop quality goals for each customer group. These were finalized in the July 1996 meeting and forwarded to the resource group for integration into the roll-out plan.

Other major action items discussed during the monthly meetings from May through July 1996 included:

- Budget for QI.
- A model for quality planning and improvement.
- Training programs for facilitators and managers,
- An electronic bulletin board to track QI activities.
- Establishment of a task force and "resource group"; as will be discussed in Steps 6 and 7, respectively.

Step 6: Task Force Meetings to Develop a QI Model and Training for Managers and Facilitators

A task force was established following the May 1996 meeting with the charge of designing a QI training program for managers (the "management toolbox"), as well as a concept paper on use and training of facilitators, and selection or design of a model for QI planning and improvement. This task force consisted of representatives from the quality, human resources, planning, education, and training offices, as well as managers from two large departments.

The group meet for three four-hour periods during the months of May and June. At the July 1, 1996, meeting of the QC, the products of the task force were presented and approved. A brief description of how each of three products was developed is provided below:

Management toolbox.

The need for a set of management skills, particularly to plan and improve quality, was initially identified in the quality assessment. These and other skills and attitudes needed by Optima managers were discussed at QC meetings, then provided to the Task Force for further consideration and development of a curriculum for the course. The results were the toolbox curriculum (Appendix C) and a model that integrated the course with other training and development efforts at Optima as shown in Figure 7.3.

Concept paper on facilitators and facilitator training.

In their deliberations, the QC identified an expanded need for facilitators for three reasons: (1) New TQM teams would be formed as a result of revitalization of the quality effort. (2) The organization was moving more towards a team-based, patient-centered approach. (3) New work groups, task forces, and transition teams were to be formed as a result of merger activities. Recognizing these and other needs, the task force drafted the concept paper as found in Appendix D.

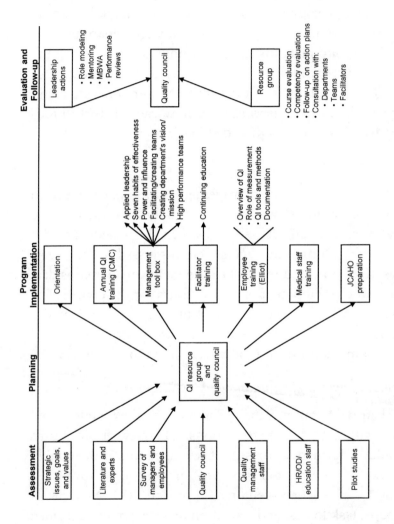

Figure 7.3 Quality Improvement Training and Development

QI model

Various strategic planning models were considered by the quality council at the April retreat and at the May meeting. The following were forwarded for consideration by the task force:

- Baldrige Award Health Care Pilot Criteria Framework (Figure 2.1).
- McKinsey's Seven-S Model (Figure 7.4).
- JCAHO's Performance Improvement Model (Figure 7.5).
- Clinical/nursing model of assessment–planning–implementation–evaluation (also, the four stages of the QBSP model shown in Figure 1.1).

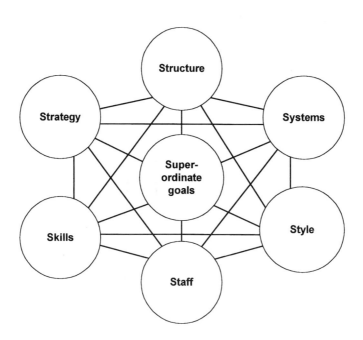

Figure 7.4 McKinsey's Seven-S Model

Source: McKinsey and Company.
Reprinted with permission.

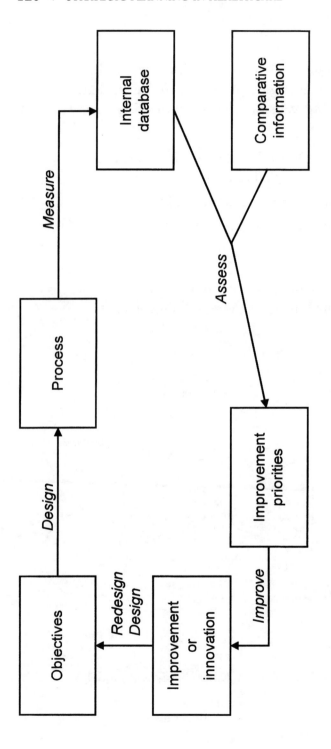

Figure 7.5 Improving Organizational Performance Function

Source: *1996 Comprehensive Accreditation Manual for Hospitals.* Oakbrook Terrace, IL: Joint Commission on Accreditation of Healthcare Organizations (1996), p. 240. Reprinted with permission.

In addition to the above, the group considered the models that were currently in use at the three major organizational entities: Juran's/Institute for Healthcare Improvement (IHI) Model at the Elliot Hospital; the JCAHO Quality Monitoring and Evaluation Model at Catholic Medical Center (CMC); and the Organization Dynamics, Inc. (ODI) Model at the Visiting Nurses Service (VNS). Each of these are displayed in Table 7.3, along with the JCAHO Performance Improvement Model.

The model recommended as the new Optima model is the clinical model shown in the first column and compared with others in remaining columns of Table 7.3. This model was selected for the following reasons: (1) It matched with the existing clinical framework of healthcare professionals. (2) It could be used for quality planning and improvement at all levels, that is, strategic/corporate, departmental, cross-functional teams, and individuals. (3) It served to unify the different models which were in use in different parts of the organization.

Step 7: Establishment of a Resource Group to Develop the QI Roll-Out Plan

During the May and June, 1996, meetings, the QC finalized the membership (see below) and the charge (roles and responsibilities) of the resource group (RG). Essentially, the RG would be the right arm of the QC, developing detailed action plans, overseeing training, starting up cross-functional teams, and conducting other activities as listed in Appendix B.

Membership of the Optima Resource Group

- VP, TQM and acute services.
- VP, human resources.
- Quality director, Elliot Hospital.

Table 7.3: Optima Health Quality Improvement Model Comparisons

Optima Model	JCAHO	Shewhart Cycle	Catholic Medical Center	Elliot Hospital/IHI/Juran	VNS/ODI Focus
Assess	**Plan** The organization has a planned, systematic, organization-wide approach to designing, measuring assessing, and improving itsperformance.	Plan	Assign responsibility. • departmental or cross-functional teams. Delineate scope of care/service. Prioritize aspects of care/functions. Identify indicators.	Assign responsibility. Delineate scope of care and service. Identify important aspects of care or service. Identify indicators.	Focus
Plan	**Design** New processes are designed well. **Measure** The organization has a systematic process in place to collect data for designing and assessing new processes, measuring and evaluation performance, identifying areas for possible improvement and determining whether changes improved the process.	Do	Establish thresholds for evaluation. Collect and organize data. Evaluate the results • analyze data to identify areas of non-conformance with thresholds. • develop a hypothesis of the root causes of the existing problem.	Establish performance triggers for evaluation. Monitor, collect, and organize data. IHI/Juran Evaluate care/service when triggered into doing so to identify the root cause(s) of the problem: • Analyze the symptoms of the problem. • Formulate theories of cause(s). • Test theories.	Analyze
Implement	**Improve** The organization systematically improves its performance.		Determine and implement appropriate action	IHI/Juran • Develop alternative solutions. • Take action to improve care/service or to correct the problem. • Deal with resistance to change. • Establish operational controls to keep performance from dropping back.	Develop Execute
Evaluate	**Assess** The organization has a systematic process to assess collected data to determine compliance with design specifications, level of compliance, priorities, actions, and the result of enacting changes to the process.	Check	Evaluate effectiveness of the action and document the level of improvement.	Assess the effectiveness of the actions taken.	
			Communicate and report relevant information.		
		Act	Continuous monitoring/improving on the process.		

- Quality director, Catholic Medical Center.
- Director, organization development.
- Director, education.
- Director, planning.
- Director, patient services.
- Representative, visiting nursing services.
- Representative, regional cardiac institute.
- Representative, marketing.
- Representative, finance.
- Representative, medical staff.

Using the outline for the roll-out plan found in Chapter 3 (page 50) and the quality objectives set by the QC, the resource group is now developing specific action plans. This roll-out plan will thus be the roadmap for quality improvement at Optima.

Sisters of Charity: An Example of the Integration of Quality Improvement and Strategic and Financial Planning

Background/Overview

The basic model or process used by the Sisters of Charity of the Incarnate Word Health Care System to integrate QI planning, strategic planning, and financial planning is called "Customer-Driven Strategic Planning" (Figure 7.6).

The model was developed and tested over a four-year period beginning in 1990 at the Sisters of St. Mary's (SSM) Health Care System based in St. Louis. The effort at SSM was coordinated by Gayle Capozzalo who served as senior vice president-strategic development. Ms. Capozzalo is currently the senior vice president of organizational development at the Sisters of Charity Health Care System (SCHCS).

SCHCS, headquarted in Houston, Texas, is a system consisting of eight hospitals, three nursing homes, physician practices, medical services organizations (MSOs), and HMOs in four states (Texas, Arkansas, Louisiana, and Utah) and in Ireland. In 1994, the leaders at SCHCS adapted and deployed the SSM model, focusing on the following features and principles:

1. Determination of customer and community needs.
2. Consideration of the organization as a system consisting of interrelated parts and processes
3. Explicit consideration of vision and values.
4. Strategic planning prior to financial planning.
5. Identification of a few, key strategic goals.
6. Deployment of strategic goals to operations (departments).
7. Initiation of improvement projects (QI teams) based on strategic goals.
8. Involvement of managers, clinicians, and line staff.
9. Ease of monitoring and updating the plan.
10. Applicability to any organizational level.

The Organization as a System

The foundation for Steps 1 and 2 of the model is the organization as a system (OAS) concept developed by Deming (1994). As seen in Figure 7.7, the concept reflects the assertion that organizational success is based on addressing three basic concerns (Batalden and Stolz, 1994):

1. How do we make what we make?
2. Why do we make what we make?
3. How can we improve what we make?

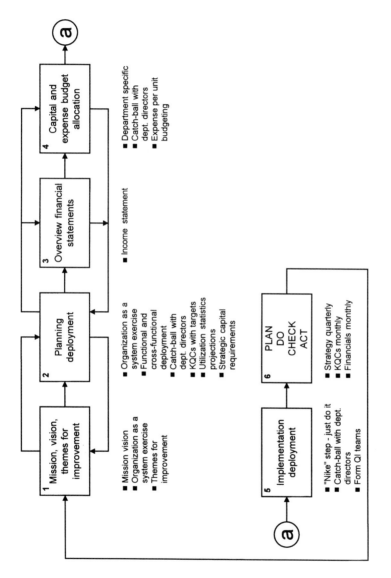

1 Mission, vision, themes for improvement
- Mission vision
- Organization as a system exercise
- Themes for improvement

2 Planning deployment
- Organization as a system exercise
- Functional and cross-functional deployment
- Catch-ball with dept. directors
- KQCs with targets
- Utilization statistics projections
- Strategic capital requirements

3 Overview financial statements
- Income statement

4 Capital and expense budget allocation
- Department specific
- Catch-ball with dept. directors
- Expense per unit budgeting

5 Implementation deployment
- "Nike" step - just do it
- Catch-ball with dept. directors
- Form QI teams

6 PLAN DO CHECK ACT
- Strategy quarterly
- KQCs monthly
- Financials monthly

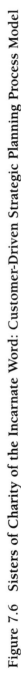

Figure 7.6 Sisters of Charity of the Incarnate Word: Customer-Driven Strategic Planning Process Model

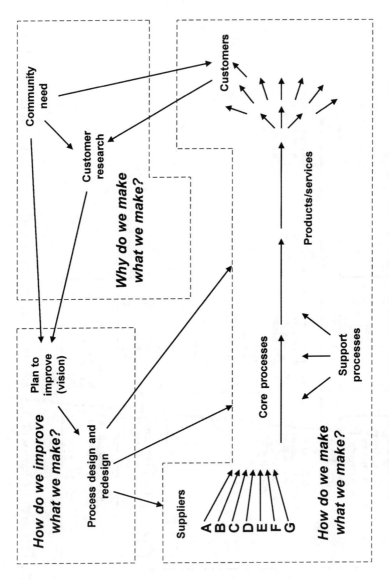

Figure 7.7   Sisters of Charity of the Incarnate Word: The Organization as a System

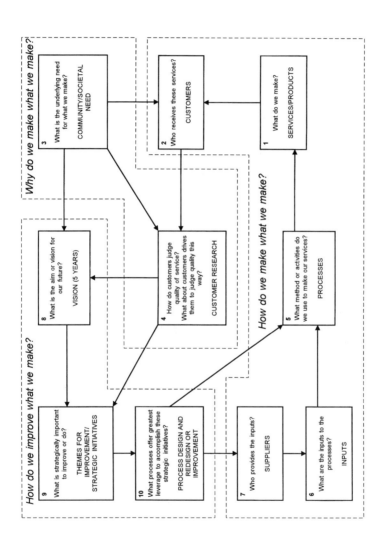

Figure 7.8 Step 1 and 2: The Organization as a System Analysis Tool

Table 7.4: The Organization as a System—Key Questions and Actions

Question 1:	**What do we make? (services/products)**
Key action:	Review of current vision, mission, and values, resulting in a statement of the core services/products that the organization provides.
Question 2:	**Who receives these services? (customers)**
Key action:	Identification of key customer groups (patients, families, the community, and physicians).
Question 3:	**What is the underlying need for what we make? (community/social need)**
Key actions:	a. Assessment of health status; demographic, epidemiologic, and utilization trends; needs of businesses; and extent, capabilities, and linkages among community services.
	b. Input from community leaders at strategic planning retreats and the community at large through focus groups at community centers, religious organizations, etc.
	c. Identification of needed services not being provided or emphasized in the community (the gaps in care or delivery of service).
Question 4:	**How do customers judge quality of service? What drives customers to judge quality this way? (customer research)**
Key actions:	a. Review of focus groups, satisfaction surveys, and market research results.
	b. Identification of key quality characteristics (KQCs) and the "drivers" for each customer group (what is important to each customer and why) through use of the nominal group and multi-voting techniques.
	c. Brainstorming of innovative services that address the drivers for each customer group.
Question 5:	**What method or activities do we use to make our services? (processes)**
Key action:	Identification of core and support processes for each service/product identified in question 1 and potential services identified in question 4.

Questions 6 and 7: What are the inputs and suppliers to the processes? (inputs and suppliers)

Key actions: a. Determination of who provides inputs or affects organizational processes (e.g., physicians, employees, vendors, payers, government).

b. Analysis of medical staff (e.g., specialties, age, their strategic plans, admission/utilization trends).

c. Technology assessment (e.g., possible new equipment, procedures, drugs and their financial and reimbursement implications; as well as ethical and moral issues).

d. Environmental/future assessment (e.g., health-care regulation, reimbursement, managed care).

e. Internal assessment (e.g., strong and weak services; benchmark comparisons with competitors on cost, price, quality, and efficiency; trends in performance indicators; and needs and expectations of employees and vendors, etc.).

Question 8:   **What is the aim or vision for our future? (five-year vision)**

Key actions: a. Consideration of customer needs, other market research, and corporate mission, vision, values, and strategic initiatives.

b. Determination of vision through an exercise in which individuals (via brainstorming) and then small groups (via affinity diagramming) come to agreement on statements in a hypothetical national magazine article that is written about the organization five years in the future. The headers of the affinity diagram are prioritized and a vision/mission statement (sometimes called the aim) is drafted.

Question 9:   **What is strategically important to improve or do? (themes for improvement/strategic initiatives)**

Key actions: a. Brainstorming of ideas by asking: "What initiatives need to be accomplished in the next three years that would have the greatest impact on our customers?

b. ˋConsolation and prioritization of ideas, resulting in no more than three themes for improvement (also called strategic initiatives or goals).

The OAS concept was adapted by SCHCS into a tool for strategic quality planning (Figure 7.8). As seen, the tool consists of a series of ten questions which relate and build upon each other.

The leaders at SCHCS determined that the OAS concept and tool directly supported the principles identified earlier. The OAS concept showed the relationships among key elements, such as the linkage of vision, community needs, customer needs, and organizational processes. Thus, participation in an OAS exercise would create a greater understanding of these relationships and the systems nature of the organizations (e.g., that if one optimizes any part of the system, one does so to the detriment of the others).

To conduct the planning effort, a strategic planning team was formed at the facility consisting of all senior leaders and representatives from the board of directors and the medical staff. The team answered questions 1 through 8 in a series of meetings or off-site retreats. Department directors were brought into the process by being asked to respond to the vision drafted by the strategic planning team (during question 8). Department directors then continued with the team in answering questions 9 and 10.

The six steps of the Customer-Driven Strategic Planning Model (Figure 7.6) will be discussed below, including the specific issues or questions addressed within each step.

Step 1: Mission/Vision and Themes for Improvement

Questions 1 through 9 are addressed in Step 1, resulting in a mission/vision statement and themes for improvement. Table 7.4 describes the key actions that occur for each question.

Step 2: Planning Deployment

As one can see in Figure 7.9, Step 2 takes the vision and themes for improvement generated from Step 1 and converts these into more specific, concrete actions.

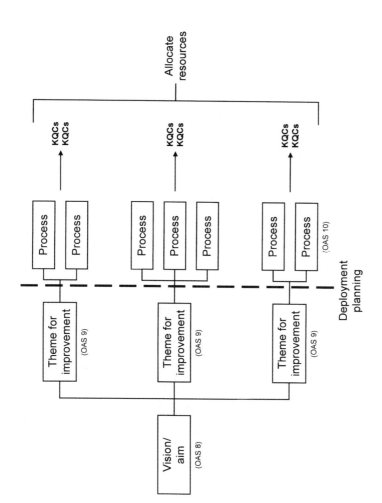

Figure 7.9 Step 2: Deployment—From Abstract to Concrete

The key actions taken within Step 2 are as follows:

1. Review of strategic initiatives (themes of improvement), brainstorming the answer to Question 10 (the last question in the OAS exercise): What processes offer the greatest leverage to accomplish these strategic initiatives? (A follow-up question is: What should we target to enhance, rearrange, redesign, eliminate, etc., to complete each initiative?)

2. Prioritization of the responses to result in identification of two or three processes per strategic initiatives based on impact and chronology (the latter being processes which need to be designed before others can begin).

3. Determination of KQC measures for each process. Thus, a measurement system (database) must be built that will provide indicators to determine the efficacy of each process.

4. Assignment of responsibility for each process. If it is a cross-functional process, then a vice president would be designated as the process "champion." A matrix diagram is used to identify those with primary and secondary responsibilities and those who need to be informed with regard to how each process is being designed, redesigned, or improved.

5. Estimation of resource requirements (from both the capital and expense budgets) to support the design, redesign, or improvement of each process.

6. Assignment of time frames for completion.

Step 3: Overview, Financial Statements

Projections of income/revenue, expenses, workload, and available capital are developed for each department, and, ultimately, for the entire organization for the next three years. This information will be used in determining allocations for capital and expense budgets.

Step 4: Capital and Expense Budget Allocation

Each capital request must show how it meets the needs of customers and/or addresses the strategic initiatives. Capital requests are classified in one of three categories. The categories and their order of priority are:

1. Safety and code (capital expenditures to ensure the safety of patients, physicians, employees, and other customers and/or to comply with codes or regulations).

2. Strategic (capital expenditures to address processes that have been targeted for design, redesign, or improvement). If insufficient capital is available for all processes, then the most important ones are fully funded rather than distributing available capital among all processes which almost always results in no one process being completed satisfactorily.

3. Infrastructure (capital expenditures that are not safety/code or strategic, such as updates to the management information system, clinic expansions, etc.).

Expense budgets for each department are negotiated by department directors with the vice presidents based on cost per "unit of service" in each department. (The unit of service is a utilization indicator that is based on workload data.) Department directors are then given a total budget for their department, rather than a budget for different expense items such as salaries, supplies, and professional development. Hence, directors have autonomy for managing an overall budget and can quickly allocate resources to areas for improvement or development as needed.

Finally, the organization sets aside an expense budget for those processes being designed, redesigned, or improved. This budget would be maintained as a part of the organization's administration budget.

Step 5: Implementation Deployment

The organization now has a strategic plan. From the previous four steps, it has defined its vision/mission; determined its strategic initiatives; identified processes (that need to be designed, redesigned or improved); and established measures, responsibilities, and budgets. Now it is time to carry out the plan.

During implementation, two critical activities must occur. The first is the deployment of the cross-functional teams to work on the processes that affect multiple departments. The second is leadership of, and communication among, the VPs and department directors with regard to changes and improvement projects within the department.

Step 6: Plan, Do, Check, Act

The Shewhart Cycle (plan, do, check, act) clearly suggests that the organization check on its plans and deployment of those plans and then take action as needed. Accordingly, SCHCS carries out the following:

1. Review of entire plan on a quarterly basis.
2. Monitoring of all measures (KQCs) on a monthly basis.
3. Financial analysis of capital and expense budgets on a monthly basis.

Time Frames and Results

Figure 7.10 provides the timeline for the strategic planning effort at SCHCS.

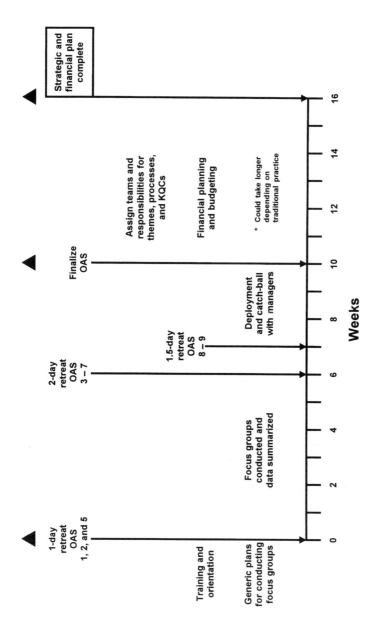

Figure 7.10 Typical Timeline for Strategic Planning Using the Organization as a System Tool

Based on the experience of Gayle Capozzalo, who led planning efforts at SSM and the Sisters of Charity Health Care Systems, the following were identified as the key benefits and lessons learned.

- Linkage of resource requirements to strategic initiatives. One member of an planning team has said: "When we used to do strategic planning, we'd say, 'I have $3 million, how do I spend it?' Today, we ask, 'How do I determine and meet the needs of my community and my customers, and what dollars will it take to do that?'"

- Greater understanding and commitment by directors and managers to the strategic plan since they all participated through the process of catch-ball.

- Greater understanding that the organization is a complicated system requiring considerable cooperation among departments to ensure that processes are well designed and meet the needs of customers.

- Alignment of quality teams and other quality efforts with the strategic initiatives of the organization; hence, management, the workforce, and the board make certain that quality improvement efforts have value and that the organization is receiving the "greatest bang for their buck."

- When a major change is made, such as the strategic and financial planning process, it takes time and dedicated effort to clearly articulate the rationale for change.

- The new strategic planning process must show clear benefits, including time savings over the previous process, to be accepted.

- The plan-do-check-act cycle gives participants time to understand and become committed to the process.

- The strategic planning process requires considerable trust between the corporate office and member organizations. Corporate offices should only set general parameters; each member organization should be entrusted to research and understand its local environment. As a result, the leadership level changes from setting direction and checking results to facilitating and coaching as the member organization gains experience with the planning process.

- The "organization as a system" exercise requires excellent facilitation.

- The planning process requires that all participants be familiar with, and committed to, TQM principles.

- All participants must understand and be able to utilize the following tools: organization as a system, affinity diagram, responsibility matrix, and the interrelationship diagram.

- Catch-ball takes time and effort; the department directors and managers must change their roles from supervisors to partners.

- Finally, departments (such as radiology and laboratory) that traditionally have been revenue generating are no longer identified as such because only expenses are budgeted. Therefore, previous relationships regarding priority of capital change, causing discomfort among directors and managers. Senior leaders must use coaching skills to mentor these directors and managers through this new paradigm (changing from a revenue center to an expense center). This is particularly crucial as managed care and capitation contracts force organizations to reduce; utilization of all services. (Sources: Capozzalo, 1993; interviews with the author July, 1996.)

Walter Reed Army Medical Center: A Case Example of the Integration of the Strategic Planning and TQM Functions

Background

This case example will focus on the strategic planning process undertaken by Walter Reed Army Medical Center (WRAMC) during the period from December 1991 through August 1993. During this twenty-month period, the author served as the director of strategic planning and TQM. The discussion will also address follow-up efforts and changes to strategic planning and TQM at Walter Reed from August 1993 to the time of publication.

WRAMC is a 600-bed academic medical center in Washington, D.C. that provides care in 68 sub-specialties to military beneficiaries who mainly reside in the north-eastern part of the US or in Europe. In late 1991, the organization embarked on a process that integrated the TQM and strategic planning processes. During the previous 18 months, both functions had been relatively dormant. Top leadership determined that it would be best to combine and revitalize both functions for the following five reasons:

1. There was a lack of integration of plans and clear strategic focus for the Medical Center since previous strategic planning largely consisted of a roll-up of departmental plans.

2. Strategic planning and TQM were viewed as key and inter-related methods to effect change in the organization, particularly to integrate plans from very diverse and autonomous departments.

3. TQM teams and other efforts would be aligned strategically.

4. Consolidation of strategic planning and TQM under one office would save organizational resources.

5. There was the strong belief and desire on the part of the commander (director) of WRAMC that all planning should be rooted in TQM philosophy with its emphasis on empowerment, participation, and customer orientation.

The Process

Overview

TQM was viewed as part of the strategic planning process, not separate from it. Thus, the overall process was labelled "strategic planning" as seen in Figure 7.11. One steering council (SC) provided oversight for both strategic planning and TQM.

Steering Council and the TQM Infrastructure

As listed before in Table 3.2, the steering council consisted of the following members:

- Director of clinical services (chair).
- Chief operating officer.
- Chief, Department of Medicine.
- Chief, Department of Surgery.
- Chief, Department of Nursing.
- Director of strategic planning and TQM.

The SC reported to the executive committee of WRAMC, which was chaired by the medical center commander and consisted of the same members as the SC, except for the director of strategic planning and TQM.

To assist the SC in overseeing the TQM initiatives, a production team was formed that consisted of the following members:

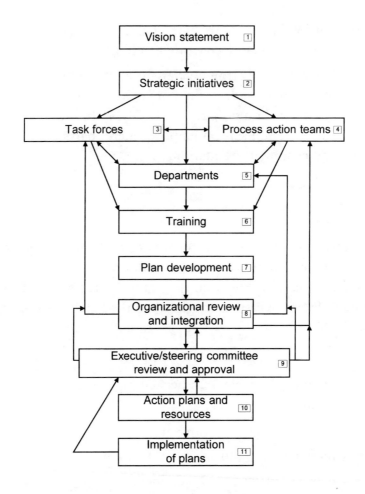

Figure 7.11   Walter Reed Army Medical Center: Strategic Planning Process

- Director of strategic planning/TQM (chair).
- Assistant director, strategic planning/TQM.
- Director of quality assurance/risk management.
- Director of clinical quality improvement.
- Director of nursing QI.
- Representative, managed care office.
- Representative, education/training office.

As seen in Figure 7.13, the production team provided direct oversight to the process action teams and coordinated quality improvement activities with departments. Additionally, the production team received quality improvement ideas from individuals throughout the organization.

After the steering council was formed in January 1992, it focused on three areas: (1) development of the strategic planning process; (2) strategic initiatives; and (3) formation of mechanisms to insure that initiatives were carried out in the organization. Later, the emphasis of the steering council was on the start-up of TQM teams and training to support strategic initiatives. Then the focus of the SC shifted to the review of plans and reports on progress from cross-functional teams, task forces, and the departments.

Below is a description of each of the 11 key elements or steps of the strategic planning process at WRAMC.

Step 1: Vision statement.

A vision statement was initially drafted by the executive committee, then distributed to the entire organization for comment over a two-month period. Input was received and consolidated by the production team, then given to the executive committee for finalization. The result is the vision statement found in Figure 7.12.

We will be the leader among healthcare institutions in the Department of Defense for healthcare, training, research, and work climate.

We will be the institution most concerned for those we serve, most chosen for the quality of our service, and most highly regarded for the excellence and commitment of our people.

We will realize our vision by being people friendly, utilizing creativity and innovative change to continually improve the services we provide.

Figure 7.12 Walter Reed Army Medical Center: Statement of Vision

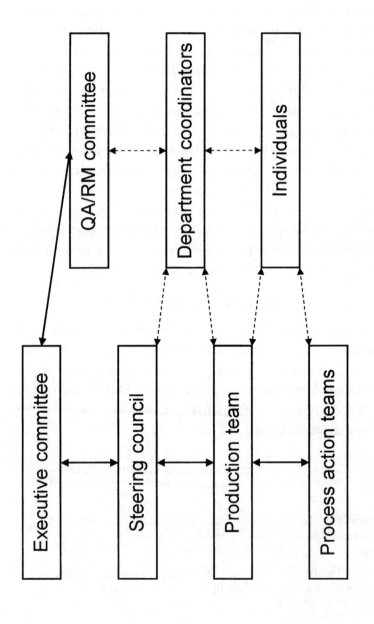

Figure 7.13   Walter Reed Army Medical Center: Quality Improvement Infrastructure

Step 2: Strategic initiatives

After the vision statement was completed, a four-hour meeting was held, attended by the steering council and the department chairs. The vision statement was posted and one question was asked: "What is getting in the way of achieving our vision?"

This question resulted in the generation of many excellent ideas, which were consolidated by affinity diagramming into the following seven categories:

1. Patient needs and expectations.
2. Graduate medical education.
3. Medical–military readiness.
4. System integration (integration of two community hospitals).
5. Work climate.
6. Organizational enhancement.
7. New/alternative mechanisms for care.

These categories became the foundation for the strategic initiatives of the organization, upon which departmental plans and TQM efforts were based and focused.

Step 3: Task forces.

A task force was established for each of the seven strategic initiatives. Each task force was provided a facilitator who was trained in TQM concepts and tools. The task force had the responsibility of reviewing all ideas from the four-hour meeting in which the strategic initiatives were established. From this review, they recommended follow-up actions to be taken by process action teams, departments, or cross-functional work groups consisting of representatives from affected departments.

Once the work groups were formed, the task forces were abolished. In effect, the task forces were replaced by the work groups, which addressed specific issues, and by the steering council, which provided general oversight of the strategic planning process.

Step 4: Process action teams.

The task forces sent recommendations for process action teams (or PATs) to the production team for consideration. The production team reviewed these recommendations along with numerous ideas from department managers and employees throughout the organization. The production team consolidated these ideas and prioritized them according to the following criteria:

- Fit with the strategic initiatives.
- Impact on patient care.
- Enhancement of patient satisfaction.

Additionally, the production team decided to limit the number of new teams to nine in order to better focus and control TQM efforts. Accordingly, the following nine teams were chartered:

1. Control of medical records.
2. Patient satisfaction survey.
3. ICU bed utilization/flow.
4. Pre-admission process.
5. Blood bank specimen labeling.
6. Nutritional assessment.
7. Radiology film tracking.
8. Control of mobile, high-value equipment.
9. Patient accommodations.

Step 5: Departments.

In addition to the planning undertaken by individual departments, the task forces identified a series of cross-functional issues which required action by multiple departments.

Twenty-six issues were identified by the task forces and subsequently approved for action planning by the steering council. These included the establishment step-down units, an ER holding area, IV/phlebotomy teams, and an HIV unit. Each issue was addressed by a work group consisting of representatives of the affected departments. A work group leader was identified by the steering council. The leader chaired the group and reported back to the steering council on action plans and progress of the group.

Step 6: Training.

All training to support the planning and TQM effort was coordinated by the production team. This allowed consistency of philosophy and content among training programs.

The following were the topics presented in a four-hour workshop to all department chairs and other members of work groups prior to the commencement of work group or department planning meetings:

- Planning process at WRAMC.
- Fundamentals of managed care and business planning.
- Preparation of business plans.
- Group decision making.
- Basic TQM concepts and methods, including planning tools.

TQM training was also offered in greater depth and for a variety of staff as outlined in Table 7.5.

Table 7.5 CQI/TQM Training Programs

Program	Length	Remarks
Awareness training	1 hour	Overview of CQI concepts and CQI program at Walter Reed. Provided at briefings and employee orientations.
Basic course	1 day	CQI concepts, problem-solving tools, team skills, and application of CQI in the daily work environment.
Executives/managers	3 days	Same as above. Additional emphasis on team-building, interdepartmental relations, CQI program implementation, and systems and process change.
Teams (just-in-time)	4 hours	Team meeting skills and techniques, group effectiveness, action planning, and statistical process control. Held immediately proper to the first team meeting.
Facilitators/trainers	5 days	All of the above plus facilitation and training techniques, meeting simulations, and feedback by instructor and peers. Co-training and facilitation required prior to "certification."
Customer service	1 day	Interpersonal skill-building in such areas as communicating with patients; managing conflict; and handling problems; inquiries and complaints through intensive role playing. Includes the Myers-Briggs Indicator.
Interpersonal skills for clinicians	4 hours	As above, but geared to the nursing and medical staff.

Step 7: Plan development.

Plans for departments were developed as outlined on pages 68-70. Important aspects of these plans included alignment with the strategic initiatives and participation of all managers within each department.

As mentioned earlier, the task forces reviewed the strategic initiatives and identified follow-on actions by the organization. These actions were then translated by the work groups into action plans, which became the essence of the strategic plan.

Finally, the process action teams developed plans for how they would proceed with process improvement. These plans would be forwarded to the production team, and then the steering council, for approval.

Step 8. Organization review and integration.

Plans from the departments and the task forces were presented and discussed at a three-day retreat attended by all senior management, department chairs, and task force leaders. The purpose of the retreat was threefold:

1. To obtain feedback on the efficacy of the plans. (Attendees provided comments in open session, then evaluated each plan on a one-to-five scale.)

2. To integrate plans based on an assessment of the impact of each plan on other departments and the total effect of all plans on the organization.

3. To create a base of support ("buy-in") for the resulting strategic plan.

Step 9. Executive committee/steering council review and approval.

The steering council reviewed all input that was provided at the retreat. In addition, the steering council received reports from the leaders of the process action teams and the work groups. Based on all this information, the steering council recommended a strategic plan which was ultimately approved by the executive committee.

Step 10. Action plans and resources.

The steering council notified the departments, work groups, and process action teams of the strategic plan and required each to submit action plans and resource requirements to the council. These action plans and resource requirements were then reviewed by the steering council and forwarded for final approval, including budget allocations, by the executive committee.

Step 11. Implementation of plans.

Plans were then implemented by the departments, work groups, and process action teams. Review of progress was assessed by the steering council and the executive committee as follows:

- Departments—review of the status of plans and workload data at the quarterly review and analysis meeting attended by all department chairs.

- Process action teams—monthly written reports of progress (limited to one page) to the production team and the steering council; and quarterly presentations to the steering council.

- Work groups—monthly reports to the steering council and quarterly meetings of team leaders with the steering council.

Recent Changes to Strategic Planning and TQM

A new committee structure was put in place at WRAMC on September 1, 1995 (see Figure 7.14).

As shown, the Governing Body replaced the Executive Committee. Membership was the same, except that two voting members were added: the director for medical administration and operations, and the command sergeant

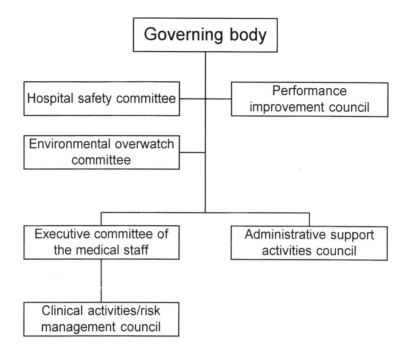

Figure 7.14   Walter Reed Army Medical Center:
New Committee Structure

major (who represented the large number of the military staff members).

In addition, three consultants attended the meetings as non-voting members: the director of clinical performance improvement and risk management (who assumed former responsibilities from the director of strategic planning and TQM), the director of patient administration, and the director of resource management.

These five additions allowed for greater consideration of issues as they affect patients, employees, and resources.

Also, as seen in Figure 7.14, the performance improvement council (PIC) replaced both the steering council and the production team. This change was made because the production team had accomplished its mission regarding the revitalization of the strategic planning and TQM processes, including the start-up of process action teams and the development of TQM training programs.

As shown below, the members of the PIC now reflect a broader cross-section of the organization:

- Director, Department of Medicine (chair).
- Director of clinical performance improvement and risk management.
- Three chairs from the medical staff departments.
- Three chairs from the administrative departments.
- Nursing quality improvement coordinator.
- Representative from the medical administration and operations office.
- Senior representative from the military staff.

Finally, in mid 1996, WRAMC reexamined the vision statement shown in Figure 7.13. The result was a more comprehensive statement that included four key elements as seen in Appendix A: mission, vision, values, and command philosophy. These four elements are now being used as the basis for a new strategic plan and as guidance for all departments and process action teams.

CHAPTER 8

CONCLUSIONS AND LESSONS LEARNED

Based on the review of the case studies, other literature, and the experience of the author, the following is a summary of conclusions and lessons learned regarding quality-based strategic planning in healthcare.

✓ *1. Have a model or road-map to follow.*

To conduct strategic planning, a model or process to focus and guide efforts is needed. Different models or approaches were presented in the case studies—all of which work for their own organizations. However, all have three critical elements in common:

1. A focus on customers, particularly assessment of needs and expectations.

2. Linking of quality plans to strategic initiatives.

3. Ongoing review and continuous quality improvement.

Organizations undertaking strategic planning can select among these models, develop their own models, or use a synthesis of different models. The selection or building of

151

a model must be based on existing culture and frameworks familiar to the organization. The four-phase strategic planning model (Assessment–Planning–Implementation–Evaluation) submitted by this author (Figure 1.1, p.11) and used at Optima Health, Inc. has the advantages of being simple and matching the existing framework of the clinical or nursing model. (A detailed step-by-step outline for use of the four-phase model can be found in Appendix F.) Additionally, it approximates the Joint Commission on Accreditation of Healthcare Organizations' performance improvement model found on page 120.

2. Develop an infrastructure for QBSP.

The key elements of an infrastructure for QBSP are a steering council (or quality council) and a resource group. Their primary functions are summarized in Table 8.1:

Table 8.1: Summary of Key Roles of the Steering Council and Resource Group

Steering Council	Resource Group
Oversee all efforts	Monitor progress of efforts
Allocate resources	Identify resource requirements
Determine vision, mission, values, guiding principles, and quality goals	Facilitate implementation of quality goals through training and consultation with departments, teams, and task forces
Approve action plans and/ or the roll-out plan	Develop action plans and/or the roll-out plan

3. Formulate a roll-out plan with timelines.

A roll-out plan with clear timelines for quality improvement efforts in the organization is critical to the realization of quality goals. Without it, key activities are forgotten or key sequential events (such as training a sufficient number of facilitators prior to the start-up of teams and task forces) do not happen. The roll-out plan, as outlined in Chapter 3 (page 50) can serve as a checklist for the steering council and resource group in overseeing or monitoring QI efforts.

4. Align core values with organizational change efforts.

To create an organizational culture for quality improvement, plans need to be formulated for a set of behaviors, attitudes, and skills. This will result in operationalizing the core values and, thus, create the climate for a learning organization.

This can best be achieved by addressing, in turn, four questions:

1. What do the values or guiding principles mean to our department, team, or task force?

2. How can we apply these values and principles to our department, team, or task force?

3. What do they mean to me as a member of the organization?

4. How can I apply them in my daily work?

A concept now frequently appearing on values statements of healthcare organizations is that of a "learning community" or a "learning organization." Unfortunately, what is meant by a "learning community" or "learning organization" is not defined well by most organizations. Below are listed characteristics that can help one to identify what a "learning organization" would look like. As part of the planning process, these characteristics could be translated into goals or additional guiding principles.

Characteristics of a Learning Organization

- Responsiveness to customers.
- Managers and employees are willing to take risks.

- Communication fully occurs up, down, and across the organization.
- Feedback is used for both individual growth and organizational change.
- Workers feel like owners.
- Everyone is a leader.
- Workers trust each other and treat each other with respect.
- The organization benefits from lessons learned.
- Core values of the organization are supported by beliefs, assumptions, behavior, skills, and organizational structure.
- Mechanisms are available for continuous learning throughout the organization.

5. Lead the effort.

Leading QBSP requires many things. The three most important leadership actions are:

1. Leading by "walking the talk," role modeling, and rewarding the desired behaviors which are expected by all members of the organization. This would include making quality improvement an agenda item at all staff meetings.

2. Obtaining feedback on leadership behavior and strategic planning initiatives. This can best be achieved by one-on-one feedback by a consultant or a trusted peer or mentor. Additionally, the steering council should collectively reflect and obtain feedback on its actions from the resource group as well as department managers.

3. Removing barriers, allocating resources, and providing time so that departments, teams, and indi-

viduals have the capacity to plan and carry out quality improvement activities.

Unless leaders carry out the above, QBSP will be considered a fad—the management flavor of the month.

6. Identify internal champions and change agents.

Consultants can clearly provide much valuable momentum and expertise to start the strategic planning process. However, between visits of the consultant and, particularly, after the consultant permanently leaves, it is crucial to have internal champions and change agents to ensure the process does not falter and the momentum continues. These individuals usually come from the five sources: top management, the steering council, the resource group, the HRD or OD departments, and informal leaders in the organization. These individuals serve in three vital capacities: "walking the talk," planning specific implementation approaches, and overcoming resistance and other barriers to strategic planning.

7. Give QBSP the time it deserves.

There are three problems with respect to time and QBSP:

1. Waiting for the "right time for strategic planning." A refrain frequently heard by this writer is: "We'll begin right after the JCAHO survey, summer vacations, Christmas, merger talks, _____." (Fill in the blank as appropriate.)

2. Allowing daily operations, crises, and "other more immediate priorities" to take precedence over strategic planning and improvement activities. This results in a lack of sufficient time at steering council meetings, poor attendance at team meetings or

training, or not "walking the talk" in the departments and on the nursing units.

3. Demanding immediate and positive results. These
demands can create an environment that precludes
sufficient time for planning and implementing
change, learning from experiences, and making
corrective actions to QI plans. If this environment
exists and QBSP results are not positive and immediate, the organization often reverts back to old
patterns and behaviors such as top-down planning,
a hierarchal structure, threats, etc.

Clearly, organizations are experiencing ongoing change.
The metaphor used by Vaill (1989 and 1996) of "managing
in permanent white water" seems to be consistent with the
healthcare environment today. Thus, managers at all levels
must allocate time for reflective thought—to ask why
things are so chaotic and busy, to identify the barriers to
quality of care and service, to review the results of quality
activities, and to prepare for change accordingly.

8. Make some things mandatory.

In an ideal world, managers and staff would be eager to
fully embrace QI initiatives—planning; scheduling themselves for all QI classes; volunteering for process action
teams and task forces; and identifying opportunities at
every turn. All this might occur, but not immediately. A
culture must first be created with the characteristics of the
learning organization as identified above.

When management initiatives are optional, participation in planning activities tends to be limited due to press-
ing operational demands, so training often results in
"preaching to the choir."

The following areas should be mandatory due to their
importance to the SQP effort:

- Planning in each department.
- QI training for all managers and employees.
- Just-in-time training for teams.

9. Make everyone a quality leader.

Senge (1990) considers the assumption that only top management can cause significant change "deeply disempowering." Managers of departments or services—cardiac institutes, cancer centers, and departments of medicine and nursing all have influence over large numbers of staff—and can effect major quality improvements. Additionally, all individuals can be leaders, plan for changes in their area of work, and make a difference, particularly if their efforts are combined with those of others who share a commitment to quality improvement.

10. Set up teams for success.

The steering council and the resource group should insure that the following ingredients for team success are present:

- Linkage of team objectives to the strategic imperatives or issues of the organization.
- Judicious selection of team members, a facilitator, and a team leader.
- A clear charter and problem statement, and target dates for interim reports and completion of activities.
- Team-building and training in QI methods.
- Coordination of the each team's activities with those of other teams and departments.

11. Set up training for success.

The following elements were found to be critical in the design and conduct of training in support of QBSP efforts:

- Design of a total system of development as shown in Figure 7.3, beginning with the assessment of needs and concluding with evaluation, follow-up, and reinforcement of learning.
- Integration of the key organizational topics of quality improvement, cost reduction, and service excellence.
- Linkage to and integration of all training programs to ensure a common language, definitions, messages, and models; avoid duplication of training material; and supplement and reinforce what is being taught in other courses.
- Conduct of training using adult learning principles— experiential exercises, interactive lectures, and group discussion on issues of relevance to the participants.
- Use of the training as an opportunity for top managers to meet and discuss issues with participants, define expectations, impart values, and even to teach part of the subject matter.
- Provision of just-in-time training, particularly, for teams, so that training can be immediately applied and thus reinforced.

12. Continually review, improve, and learn.

In the final phase of QBSP strategic planning (evaluation and CQI), the following are deemed to be most important:

- Revisit all quality goals at each steering council or resource group meeting.
- Establish and maintain a "dashboard" of key measures.
- Have quality improvement as a specific agenda item at each staff meeting—continually address what can be done to enhance the care, service, or value to our

consumers. Eventually, this agenda item creates an awareness that results in every member of the staff looking for ways to improve quality as part of their daily work.

- Disseminate knowledge gained from quality improvement activities by establishing such mechanisms as quality days or forums, liaisons or "internal networkers" (Senge, 1994) to move ideas across the organization to other teams and departments, "journal clubs" on concepts and cases from the literature, or discussion groups in which lessons from QI activities are shared.

13. Use a quality coach or consultant, but limit their role.

The consultant, sometimes called the "quality coach," can be extremely valuable to the organization by:

- Generating interest and validating the need for QBSP for "no man is a prophet in his own land."
- Providing expertise, particularly in the various options of models and approaches, as well as first-hand experience in what has worked or has not worked in other healthcare organizations.
- Conducting training, running team-building sessions, and facilitating the initial meetings of the steering council and the resource group.
- Reviewing quality goals, drafts of the roll-out plan, action plans, training curricula, and policies describing the process for strategic planning in the organization.
- Providing candid feedback to the organization on the QBSP efforts and the actions/behavior of top manage-

ment, the steering council, the resource group, trainers, and facilitators. This "mirror of observations" can be extremely valuable in allowing the organization to see itself as it goes through the strategic planning process.

Clearly, consultants can provide considerable value to the strategic quality planning process; however, a few cautions or "don'ts":

- Do not rely too heavily on the consultant, as this may create a dependency on part of the key members involved with the strategic planning process. Because of time constraints, there is a strong tendency to have the consultant do work than could be done more cost-effectively (e.g., documentation of meetings) or more appropriately by the organization.

- Do not use the consultant's strategic planning model or process without critical reviews by the steering council, resource group, and departments.

- Do not have the consultant do all the thinking. Think with the consultant to develop an understanding of the concepts, methods, and implementation approaches. Evaluate the consultant's ideas and take time to adapt them to the unique situation and culture of the organization, playing catch-ball with these ideas with the steering council, resource group, and the departments. The organization will then develop its own model and approaches, thereby creating a more acceptable and workable strategic planning process.

APPENDIX A

MISSION, VISION, AND VALUES STATEMENTS

Optima Health

Mission

We are dedicated to improving the health and well being of our community by providing compassionate, caring and accessible health care. We affirm individual worth and dignity by addressing the needs of the mind, body and spirit.

Vision

Everything we do is guided by our mission and values. As the responsive and innovative health care leader in the region, we are recognized as a center of excellence and for the expertise of our staff. Through our commitment to providing a lifetime of care, we meet the diverse needs and exceed the expectations of our community. We take pride in our collaborative relationships with patients, employees, physicians, volunteers and other health care partners Through our dedication to health and wellness, we are creating a better community in which to work and live.

Values

We are committed to the **highest standards of quality and excellence**. We are dedicated to sustaining financial strength through the sound management of our resources. We are accountable to our community for the quality and value of the services we provide.

Open and honest communication is essential to our mission. We foster and actively promote an environment where all are free to share their ideas and concerns without fear of reprisal. We show respect for each other at all levels.

Our commitment to respect and dignity begins with our **valued employees, physicians and volunteers**. This family is nurtured in an environment marked by high standards and expectations, with opportunities for learning, mobility and growth.

We believe that pride and ownership through participation and shared responsibility creates a strong Optima Health **family**.

Creativity and innovation are key to our success. We reward employees who help us unlock the human potential that exists within our organization.

We work together as partners in a spirit of cooperation. **Collaboration** is vital to achieve our mission of caring and serving.

Walter Reed Army Hospital

Mission

- Provide quality, comprehensive health care that is cost competitive and accessible.
- Serve as a national resource for specialty care and medical issues unique in DoD and other federal agencies.
- Maintain individual and collective readiness in support of the DoD Health Care System.

- Provide research, education and training in support of the DoD Health Care System.

Vision

- Provides ready access to comprehensive health care services.
- Promotes military medical readiness.
- Supports medical education and research.

Values

- Caring: Provide responsive, caring service to internal and external customers.
- Quality: Provide the highest quality services and always consider the value of the outcomes delivered.
- Commitment: Demonstrate relentless dedication to do whatever it takes to get the job done right.
- Innovation: Empower our staff to encourage creativity and innovation.

Command Philosophy

Patient focused care and teamwork. We are partners with the patient in the delivery of care. Together, we must do what is right for the patient, not only in terms of quality, but in the environment which maintains the patient's dignity and pride. We will treat our patients the way we would like to be treated ourselves.

Uniformed Services University of Health Sciences

Mission

The Uniformed Services University of the Health Sciences is the Nation's federal health sciences university and is committed to excellence in military medicine and public health during peace and war. We provide the Nation with health professionals dedicated to career service in the Department of Defense and the United States Public Health Service and with scientists who serve the common good. We serve the uniformed services and the nation as an outstanding academic health sciences center with a worldwide perspective for education, research, service, and consultation; we are unique in relating these activities to military medicine, disaster medicine, and military medical readiness.

Vision

We are the Nation's federal health sciences university, recognized as an outstanding scholarly educational center. Our component schools and institutes are dedicated to excellence and innovation in education, research, and service worldwide.

We are a university that grants degrees in the health sciences at all levels, producing outstanding scientists and health care practitioners for the Nation.

We are recognized as the preeminent center for the study of military medicine, tropical diseases, disaster medicine, and adaptation to extreme environments.

We are a major coordinating center for consultation, support, and advocacy education and operational readiness training in the health sciences, throughout the careers of uniformed medical personnel.

We have a cooperative, mutually supportive and valued interaction with DoD hospitals that enhances undergraduate education, graduate medical education, research programs and patient care.

We have a partnership with the Henry M. Jackson Foundation for the Advancement of Military Medicine that enriches our scholarship and contributes to our fiscal stability and maximum development.

We attract a diverse population of qualified individuals and encourage their personal and professional development. Out students, faculty, and staff appreciate that they are essential to the work and success of each other and the University.

We are exemplary in providing access and opportunity for career development to people traditionally under-represented in medicine, science, academia and government service.

We prepare and inspire our students, faculty, and staff for a lifetime of learning, leadership, and service.

Our programs, scholarly activities, faculty, and graduates make outstanding contributions throughout the medical and scientific communities.

To provide the Nation with medical officers and scientists of character who serve the common good.

Guiding Principles

As we strive to accomplish our mission we are committed to all of the following principles. Each one represents an essential and equally important core value.

Caring

We foster an atmosphere of caring, mutual respect, courtesy, pride in work and personal development. Each member of the university community is important.

Communication

We interact and share information in a timely manner with openness, candor, and sensitivity.

Integrity

We conduct ourselves responsibly, ethically, and honestly.

Loyalty

We are dedicated to each other, the University, the Department of Defense, and the Nation.

Quality

We strive to excel through continuous quality improvement.

Scholarship

We are committed to academic freedom as fundamental to the advancement of knowledge and a lifetime of learning.

Service

We are sensitive to the needs of those we serve and are responsive to new ideas and change.

Teamwork

We value the contributions of each member of our community and work to achieve an environment characterized by cooperation, collegiality, and an appreciation of diversity.

APPENDIX B

ROLES AND RESPONSIBILITIES OF THE RESOURCE GROUP

Charge: Functions under the direction of the quality council (QC). Members support the activities of the quality council in the following ways:

1. **Coordination of training.**

   a. Determines training needs including literature reviews and needs assessments (surveys and focus groups) for managers, employees, and physicians.

   b. Schedules trainers and participants.

   c. Arranges logistics: conference rooms, A-V equipment, and training certificates.

   d. Recommends QI books, videos, and other training materials for purchase.

   e. Evaluates training by:

   (1) Observing training.

   (2) Obtaining feedback on the course (immediate post-course evaluation).

(3) Conducting 3-6 month follow-up study of training effectiveness.

(4) Submitting input to the performance evaluation for trainers.

f. Conducts training (to maintain skills and creditability).

2. Liaison/coordination with teams.

a. Identifies facilitators for teams.

b. Reviews charter with team.

c. Assists in the development of the problem statement.

d. Monitors progress, identifying problems to the QC.

e. Facilitates when necessary (to maintain skills and creditability).

f. Coordinates efforts of the team with other teams, task forces, and departments.

g. Observes team meetings and evaluates the team facilitator.

h. Assists the team in preparing for presentations to the quality council.

3. Idea formulation and studies.

a. Evaluates recommendations for new QI teams.

b. Evaluates suggestions on ways to improve quality.

c. Refines and consolidates ideas for consideration by QC.

d. Recommends priorities for QI to the QC.

e. Conducts QI studies as directed by the QC.

4. Monitoring.

a. Conducts trends analysis on:

(1) Quality indicators,

(2) Patient satisfaction surveys,

(3) Employee and physician surveys and focus groups.

b. Conducts surveys and focus groups as necessary.

c. Under direction of the quality council, evaluates the overall effectiveness of the QI program.

5. **Reports.**

a. Assists teams to develop monthly and quarterly reports. Collates reports for the quality council.

b. Assists teams in keeping storyboards and story-books that reflect the work of the team.

c. Prepares the annual QI report for the quality council.

d. Under the direction of the quality council, prepares any reports for the board of directors.

e. Submits articles for internal and external publication on QI initiatives.

f. Updates the QI plan for the quality council.

APPENDIX C

THE MANAGEMENT TOOLBOX FOR QUALITY

Day 1 of the Toolbox

1. **Driving Forces** (presented by executive management team member) 8:00 A.M.–10:00 A.M.
   a. Importance of the course—need for QI and management skills.
   b. Driving forces for change (market forces, impact of managed care and third-party payers, etc.)
   c. Strategic initiatives at Optima.
   d. Role and expectations of managers:
      (1) Operationalizing organizational goals, values, and strategic initiatives.
      (2) Managing cost, quality, and customer service.
      (3) Improving employee morale.
      (4) Collaborating versus competing.

2. Quality Improvement (QI)—The Basics
10:00 A.M.–12:00 P.M.

a. Definitions: QI, TQM, CQI, and QM.

b. Critical QI concepts:

(1) Focus on the customer.

(2) The systems approach.

(3) The learning organization.

(4) Teams and teamwork.

(5) Variation, use of data, and root cause analysis.

(6) The cost of poor quality.

(7) Continuous/relentless quality improvement.

c. How QI relates to cost, operational efficiency, and utilization/case management.

d. How QI relates to service excellence.

3. QI at Optima   1:00 P.M.–2:00 P.M.

a. Optima's QI model of assessment–planning–implementation–Evaluation.

b. Quality structure at Optima.

c. Quality initiatives at Optima.

4. The Tools   2:00 P.M.–5:00 P.M.

a. Tools for group problem solving (brainstorming, nominal group, multi-voting, affinity diagramming, flow charting, root cause analysis, etc.)

b. Quantitative tools (histograms, Pareto charts, control charts, indicators, statistical process control).

c. Tools for running effective meetings (setting agendas, expectations, groundrules, dealing with difficult personalities).

Day 2 of the Toolbox

4. The Tools (continued)   8:00 A.M.–10:00 A.M.

   d. Techniques for running open forums and establishing open communication with subordinates.

   e. Tools for team-building (role clarification, responsibility charting, goal setting, evaluations for team or group effectiveness).

   f. Tools for clinical cost effectiveness (profiling, pathways, cost-effectiveness studies, trend analysis, benchmarking, etc.)

   g. Tools for assessing and using patient feedback and other customer input (employees, physicians, payers, etc.)

5. Leadership—Making Quality Happen
10:00 A.M.–12:00 P.M.

   a. Planning for quality in your department or service.

   b. Establishment of a culture/environment for quality and service excellence.

   c. Key concepts in service design, delivery, and management.

   d. Support and development for those on the front lines of care and service.

   e. Management by wandering around (MBWA), mentoring, and role modeling.

   f. Reinforcing quality training.

   g. The keys of participatory management.

   h. Change management—a primer.

   i. Situational leadership—an overview.

6. Applications and Follow-up   1:00 P.M.–5:00 P.M.

   a. Case studies.

   b. Open discussion on issues.

   c. Action plan for the implementation of key learnings.

   d. Follow-up and reinforcement of learnings.

   e. Learning resources/references (staff contacts, books, etc.).

   f. Sign up for follow-on courses (*The Seven Habits of Highly Effective People,* Situational leadership, positive power and influence, facilitating teams, etc.).

CONCEPT PAPER: FACILITATORS AND FACILITATOR TRAINING

1. Facilitators will be an organizational resource for:
   a. Cross-functional quality improvement teams (e.g., admissions process).
   b. Quality management activities.
   c. Organizational task forces.
   d. Strategic initiatives.
   e. Merger activities.
   f. Planning/project meetings.
   g. Committees and staff meetings.
   h. Town-hall meetings, focus groups, and open forums.
   i. Team-building meetings.
   j. Department activities/projects/teams (internal resource to their own departments).
   k. QI training, including just-in-time training for teams, task forces, etc.

2. Critical competencies and knowledge areas for facilitators:

　a. QI concepts.

　b. QI tools (brainstorming, nominal group, flow-charting, etc.).

　c. Statistical process control and variation.

　d. Process improvement model (including the ability to integrate previous models used at Optima).

　e. Quality structure and initiatives at Optima.

　f. Meeting management

　g. Designing and running town-hall meetings.

　h. Group dynamics.

　i. Team-building.

　j. Documentation (storyboards, storybooks, and QI reports).

3. Qualifications for selection as a facilitator:

　a. Strong interest and desire.

　b. High degree of interpersonal skills.

　c. Good record of performance in current and previous jobs.

　d. Acceptance by and creditability with peers.

　e. Approval by department director.

　f. Completion of QI basic course and facilitator's course.

4. Facilitator training:

　a. QI basic course/management toolbox—2 days.

　b. Facilitator's course—3 days.

　c. Continuing education (facilitator meetings)— 2 hrs/month.

NOTE: It is recommended that all *current* and *future* facilitators attend the new QI basic course (management toolbox) and the new facilitator's course.

5. **Target groups for facilitator training:**

   a. All QI staff.

   b. Individuals supporting merger/planning activities.

   c. Departments (at least one facilitator for each department).

   d. Physicians/medical staff leaders (3–5 physician-facilitators recommended).

   e. Management engineers.

   f. Others as designated by the QC.

6. **Summary of time commitments:**

   a. Initial training: five days (basic course plus facilitator's course).

   b. Facilitation of meetings (including preparation): no more than six hours per month as an organizational resource for cross-functional teams, merger activities, etc.

   c. Two hours per month for facilitator meetings/continuing education.

7. **How facilitators would be designated, used, and evaluated:**

   a. A memo will be sent to department directors containing the above information with request to provide a prioritized list for facilitator training. In their reply, the directors would indicate their acceptance of the time commitments found in paragraph 6. Department directors would be encouraged to select highly qualified staff.

b. The QI resource group would consolidate the lists from departments and provide an integrated, prioritized list for approval by the QC.

c. Needs for facilitators for cross-functional teams, task forces, etc. would be identified by the QI resource group. Facilitators will be provided for these and other teams/groups if the process or problem is complex, high-risk, cross-functional, or requires the use of advanced QI tools or methodologies.

d. The resource group would identify facilitators for specific teams or groups. The resource group would assess experience of the facilitator, workload of the facilitator, the nature of the problem, and team membership. Based on this assessment, the resource group would select a facilitator and notify the individual through the department director.

e. Each facilitator would have a liaison or point of contact on the resource group who will be their sponsor, providing the facilitator with assistance with team start-up, ongoing meetings, and documentation. Additionally, the sponsor will monitor the progress of the team, provide feedback to the facilitator, and submit letter of input to department director regarding their performance.

ROADMAP FOR QUALITY-BASED STRATEGIC PLANNING

Assessment Phase

A1. Establish a philosophy and structure for QBSP

a. Have a broad view or philosophy of quality improvement which includes community health status (e.g., incidence of disease), clinical quality (e.g., patient care outcomes), and service quality (e.g., admissions process, waiting times, responsiveness to third party payers).

b. Establish a steering council (SC).

    1. Role: oversee the planning process, provide direction, allocate resources, approve the plan.

    2. Members: Senior management team and the directors of quality and planning.

c. Establish a resource group (RG).

      1. Role: conduct detailed analysis, coordinate QBSP initiative efforts, oversee training and facilitation, and monitor activities.

      2. Members: selected members of the planning, quality, and HR/training staffs; along with operational representatives.

   d. Clarify roles.

      1. Quality improvement is everyone's job with every individual striving to improve quality in daily work.

      2. Department managers are owners of processes and systems, and thus ultimately accountable for process and systems outcomes.

      3. Executives and senior managers make strategic planning part of normal business since it is a standing agenda item at staff meetings.

      4. The SC and RG oversee, facilitate, and support the strategic planning process across the organization, particularly providing guidance and coordinating efforts of departments and cross-functional teams.

A2. Review and/or establish statements of vision, mission, and guiding principles (see Appendix A for examples).

   a. Establish statements based on input from across the organization.

   b. To obtain specific comments from managers and the workforce, ask the following question when they are providing ideas or reviewing drafts: "What does the vision and each of the guiding principles mean to you?"

A3. Identify key customers and assess their needs and expectations.

a. The five key customers for healthcare organizations are: patients, community, employees, physicians, and third-party payers.

b. Begin the assessment with focus groups of different customer groups to obtain in-depth knowledge, ideas for innovation, and firsthand feel of issues. Follow up with an extensive survey of all customers, particularly patients, employees, and physicians.

A4. Conduct an external assessment.

a. Examine seven key areas: health status, community resources, technology, regulation, competition, demographics, and healthcare financing.

b. Use a template to guide efforts (see External Assessment Template, page 24).

A5. Conduct an internal quality assessment.

a. Assess nine key areas: top management leadership, human resource development, medical staff, employee empowerment and teamwork, structure and infrastructure, strategic planning, customer orientation, measurement and analysis, and results.

b. Use a template such as the Internal Assessment Template (page 26), the abbreviated version (page 30), or the Malcolm Baldrige National Award Criteria.

Planning Phase

P1. Establish a philosophy for planning, emphasizing the following elements.

    a. Customers' needs and expectations, particularly those of patients, the community (health status), employees, physicians, and third-party payers.

    b. Analysis of customer needs and expectations, and market forces, to determine:

       1. Strategic goals.

       2. Focus of quality improvement (QI) projects.

    c. Catch-ball—widespread involvement and participation in the planning process by all management levels and the medical staff.

    d. Alignment of:

       1. Mission, vision, guiding principles, and goals.

       2. Strategic goals and QI projects.

       3. Quality and financial planning.

       4. Quality and cost-reduction initiatives (e.g., downsizing, restructuring, discharge planning and utilization review).

    e. Cascading of goals throughout the organization.

    f. Empowerment and accountability—giving managers and the workforce the authority and responsibility to develop and carry out goals consistent with the strategic objectives of the organization.

    g. The organization as a system—

       1. Focus on strategic interests of the overall organization.

       2. Integrate plans across the organization (avoiding suboptimization of specific functional areas or product lines).

3. Consider impacts of any goals or action plans on all parts of the organization.

P2. *Operationalize the vision statement and values.*

a. At a strategic planning retreat ask:

1. "If an article were to be written about our facility five years from now, what would you want that article to say?" This question will help people in the organization focus on (or add to) key areas in the vision statement.

2. "What does our organization need to do to realize our vision and operating values?"

3. "What is getting in the way of realizing our vision and values?"

b. During planning sessions at the department level, ask:

1. "What does the vision and values statement mean to our department?"

2. "What do we need to do, given the vision and values?"

P3. *Review the mission statement.*

a. Ensure that quality improvement is made an explicit part of the mission statement. Consider JCAHO's nine "Dimensions of Performance" as mission statement elements:

1. Efficacy.

2. Appropriateness.

3. Availability.

4. Timeliness.

5. Effectiveness.

6. Continuity of care.

7. Safety.

8. Efficiency.

9. Respect and caring.

b. Identify the implications for quality improvement
for each element of the mission statement at a
steering council meeting, then solicit additional
input from all members of the management team.

P4. Analyze internal, external, and customer/ stakeholder assessments.

a. Information from all assessments is summarized by
the resource group (RG) for consideration by the
steering council (SC).

b. The SC categorizes and prioritizes issues through
the use of affinity diagramming and multi-voting.

P5. Identify areas of improvement and key success factors (KSFs) or strategic imperatives (SIs).

a. The SC considers the following inputs:

1. Results from operationalization of the vision and
values (Step P2).

2. Results from review of the mission statement
(Step P3).

3. Internal, external, and customer/stakeholder
assessments (Step P4).

b. The SC identifies and names KSFs and SIs via
"themes for improvement" (seven or fewer, to
maintain focus and optimize resources):

1. Each member looks for themes for improvement
across all inputs.

2. Each member presents his or her recommended
themes for improvement, and the SC discusses
commonalities and differences.

3. The SC prioritizes themes by asking the key question, "Of these, what are critical to our success?" Should the group have difficulty in coming to consensus on themes, the QI tools of affinity diagramming and multi-voting are recommended.

P6. Establish quality goals.

a. Quality goals are set for each KSF or SI.

b. Criteria for quality goals:
1. Directly relate to and measure a critical aspect of each KSF or SI.
2. Directly relate to and measure critical areas of concern for each customer group (e.g., patients, physicians, employees).
3. Are measurable.
4. Focus on results rather than on activities.

c. The goals are then reviewed by the departments for their input and comment ("catch-ball").

P7. Determine quality projects.

a. Ideas for quality projects are generated by:
1. The SC and RG as they review all assessment data and identify themes for improvement (P5b).
2. Department managers as they review the KSFs, themes for improvement, and the quality goals as part of the "catch-ball" process.
3. Individuals by giving input via surveys, focus groups, and the suggestion program.

b. Evaluate and prioritize quality ideas and projects:
1. Ideas are collected and initially studied for merit by the RG.

    2. The SC reviews recommendations for projects from the RG.

    3. The SC prioritizes projects using group consensus (or multi-voting) based on the degree to which the projects support one or more of the KSFs/SIs.

c. Quality projects are forwarded to either departments (e.g., reducing ER waiting times), committees (e.g., infection control, safety), or cross-functional teams or task forces to address issues that affect many departments or services (e.g., admitting and discharge processes, patient flow through intensive care units). (Detailed information on quality projects is provided in the roll-out plan.)

P8. Develop a roll-out or implementation plan for QI.

a. Purpose: To provide a single-source document to guide the QI effort.

b. Key elements of the plan (a detailed outline of a plan from one organization is found in "Roll-Out Plan Elements" on page 50) are:

    1. Organizational philosophy of quality.

    2. Structure for quality improvement.

    3. Quality goals.

    4. QI projects.

    5. Process action teams.

    6. Departmental responsibilities.

    7. The individual's role.

    8. Measures and measurement strategy.

    9. Information systems support.

10. Training programs.

11. Use of facilitators.

12. Rewards and recognition.

13. HR, organizational development, and team-building.

14. Communications and marketing plan.

15. Evaluation of QI initiatives.

16. Resource requirements to support the plan.

c. Other parts of the plan include time frames and responsibilities for completion of each element of the plan.

d. Process: The plan is developed by the RG, reviewed by department managers, and submitted to the SC for final approval.

P9. Establish a budget.

a. Resource requirements (the last part of the roll-out plan) are carefully reviewed by the SC, of which the CFO is a member.

b. Separate appropriations may be needed to support the following resource-intensive areas:

1. Training.

2. Quality projects and benchmarking studies.

3. Rewards system.

P10. Publish and market the plan.

a. Target key groups: employees, department managers, and physicians.

b. Create communications and marketing strategies (see Table 3.4).

Implementation Phase

I1. Establish a philosophy for quality implementation, emphasizing the following principles.

 a. Quality improvement is everyone's job.

 b. Leaders/managers are owners of organizational processes and systems.

 c. There is coordination of quality initiatives across the organization ("horizontal catch-ball").

 d. Practice management-by-wandering-around (MBWA).

 e. Implementation is the hard part of quality-based strategic planning; thus considerable effort must be put into initiating actions and follow-through on plans.

I2. Executives' role.

 a. Receive training, then take part in QI training as a trainer.

 b. Be visible, "walk-the-talk," and serve as a role model for quality.

 c. Empower subordinate managers and employees to innovate and to identify QI opportunities.

 d. Align goals, values, and rewards.

 e. Recognize and reward desired behaviors.

 f. Follow up on the roll-out plan.

 g. Include QI as a specific agenda item at all staff meetings (this will keep QI on the front burner and make QI a part of daily operations).

 h. Monitor key processes—you are the owner.

i. Play catch-ball, involving your staff and coordinating initiatives across the organization.

j. Have a customer focus, constantly seeking ways to exceed needs and expectations.

13. Department managers' role.

a. Same as above.

b. Further develop key management skills (see the Management Development Program on page 71).

c. Conduct departmental planning, aligning goals with those of the organization (see example of a departmental planning process on page 68).

14. Role of each individual.

a. Seek out ways to improve quality in daily work.

b. Forward ideas to management, the RG, or the suggestion program.

c. Participate in process action teams and quality improvement projects whenever possible.

d. Attend training (see Table 4.1 for an example of training program geared to the front-line workforce).

15. Role of the cross-functional teams.

a. Carry out the charter defined by the SC.

b. Receive training as a team on the quality improvement process, problem-solving tools, and team-building.

c. Ensure that measures of success are defined.

d. Document and report results.

e. Obtain input from supervisors and fellow workers prior to team meetings and keep them informed of team progress.

16. Role of the resource group.

  a. Assist cross-functional teams with start-up, including group membership, training, team-building, and facilitation.

  b. Monitor activities of the cross-functional teams.

  c. Coordinate efforts (includes serving as a liaison) among teams and departments.

  d. Design and conduct training programs (usually accomplished by members who have expertise in training design and delivery, such as those in areas of employee, managerial, or organizational development).

  e. Receive and initially evaluate all ideas for quality improvement projects.

  f. Assist department managers in their quality efforts.

17. Role of the Steering Council.

  a. Charter quality improvement teams.

  b. Evaluate and approve recommendations for new quality projects.

  c. Provide for and adjust resources as necessary to carry out QI projects.

Evaluation & CQI Phase

E1. Maintain a philosophy for evaluation and CQI.

  a. Quality is a "race without a finish line."

  b. Innovation and the relentless pursuit of quality allow the organization to stay ahead of the competition.

E2. *Establish a measurement "dashboard."*

a. Show measures that reflect the critical aspects of each strategic imperative, quality goal, and customer group.

b. Show measures of critical organizational processes or functions (e.g., wait times, accounts receivables, patient education).

c. Show measures that determine progress towards objectives for process action teams.

d. Show quality indicators for each department.

E3. *The SC regularly reviews the following:*

a. Results of the "dashboard" and other outcome indicators.

b. Implementation of the roll-out plan, particularly the status of strategic initiatives.

c. Progress of the process action teams and departmental plans.

d. Individuals' level of complete commitment to quality improvement (see checklist on page 93).

e. Overall cost-effectiveness of quality improvement efforts, considering a cost-of-poor quality (COC) initiative.

REFERENCES

Anders, George. "Who Pays Cost of Cut-Rate Heart Care?" *Wall Street Journal*, October 15, 1996, p. B1.

Arvantes, James C. "Integrating TQM and Strategic Planning," *The Quality Letter*, Vol. 5, No. 7, September 1993, pp. 1-12.

Austin, Charles J. *Information Systems for Hospital Administration*, 3rd ed. Ann Arbor, MI: Health Administration Press, 1988.

Bader, Barry S. *Rediscovering Quality.* Rockville, MD: Bader & Associates, 1992.

Barber, Ned. *Quality Assessment for Healthcare. A Baldrige-Based Handbook.* New York: Quality Resources, 1996.

Batalden, Paul B. and Stoltz, Patricia. "Fostering the Leadership of Continually Improving Healthcare Organization," *Quality Letter,* Vol. 6, No. 6, July–August 1994, pp. 9-15.

Bergman, Rhonda. "TQM: Merger Trailblazer?" *Hospitals & Health Networks*, Vol. 68, No. 24, December 20, 1994, pp. 44-45.

Berwick, Donald. "Continuous Improvement as an Ideal in Health Care," *New England Journal of Medicine*, Vol. 320, No. 1, January 5, 1989, pp. 53-56.

——. "Improving Community Health Status," *Quality Connection*, Vol. 2, No. 4, Fall, 1993, pp. 2-3.

"Beyond Total Quality Management and Reengineering: Managing through Processes," *Harvard Business Review*, Vol. 73, No. 5, September–October 1995, pp. 80-81.

Bigelow, Barbara and Margarete Arndt. "Total Quality Management: Field of Dreams," *Health Care Management Review*, Vol. 20, No. 4, pp. 15-25.

Boerstler, Heidi, et al. "Implementation of Total Quality Management: Conventional Wisdom versus Reality," *Hospital and Health Services Administration*, Vol. 41, No. 2, Summer 1996, pp. 143-159.

Bruno, Charles. "Big Mergers Take a Human Toll," *Network World*, Vol. 12, No. 42, October 16, 1995, p. 47.

Burda, David. "Study: Mergers Cut Cost, Services, Increase Profits," *Modern Healthcare*, Vol. 23, No. 46, November 15, 1993, p. 4.

Caldwell, Chip. *Mentoring Strategic Change in Health Care*. Milwaukee: ASQC Quality Press, 1995.

Capozzalo, Gayle. "Quality Improvement Principles Power New Strategic and Financial Planning Process," *The Quality Letter*, Vol. 5, No. 7, September 1993, pp. 13-20.

Carey, Raymond G. and Robert C. Lloyd. *Measuring Quality Improvement in Healthcare: A Guide to Statistical Process Control Applications*. New York: Quality Resources, 1995.

Carf, C. and V. Navasky. *The Experts Speak*. New York: Pantheon Books, 1984.

Carlzon, Ian. *Moments of Truth*. Cambridge: Ballinger, 1987.

Chaufournier, Roger. "The Role of TQM in Vertically Integrated Health Systems," *Quality Connection*, Vol. 3, No. 1, Winter 1994, pp. 7-9.

Coile, Russell C. Jr. "Management Teams for the 21st Century," *Healthcare Executive*, Vol. 2, No. 1, January–February 1996, pp. 10-13.

Conrad, Douglas A. and Stephen M. Shortell. "Integrated Health Systems: Promise and Performance," *Frontiers of Health Services Management*, Vol. 13, No. 1, Fall 1996, pp. 3-40.

Coughlin, Kenneth, ed. *1997 Medical Quality Management Sourcebook: A Comprehensive Guide to Key Clinical Performance Measurement and Improvement Systems.* New York: Faulkner & Gray, 1996.

Deming, W. Edwards. *The New Economics.* Cambridge: MIT, 1994.

Dranove, David and Mark Shanley. "Cost Reductions or Reputation Enhancement as Motives for Mergers: The Logic of Multi-Hospital Systems," *Strategic Management Journal*, Vol. 16, No. 1, pp. 55-74.

Dyer, William G. *Team Building: Current Issues and New Alternatives,* 3rd ed. Reading, MA: Addison-Wesley, 1995.

Emanual, Ezekiel and Linda Emanual. "What Is Accountability in Health Care," *Annals of Internal Medicine*, Vol. 124, No. 2, January 1996, pp. 229-239.

Etzioni, Amitai. "The Responsive Community: A Communitarian Perspective," *American Sociological Review,* Vol. 61, February 1996, pp. 1-11.

Farmer, Randye. "After the Courtship: Managing Merger Transitions," *Bank Management*, Vol. 72, No. 3, May–June 1996, pp. 34-36.

Federal Quality Institute. *Federal Total Quality Management Handbook*. Washington, D.C. Office of Personnel management, 1990.

Fink, Arlene. *Evaluation Fundamentals: Guiding Health Programs, Research, and Policy*. Newbury Park, CA: Sage Publications, 1993.

Fisher, Donald C. and Bryan P. Simmons. *The Baldrige Workbook for Healthcare*. New York: Quality Resources, 1996.

Fontana, Thomas A., Sandra Butcher, and Sharon Ann O'Brien. "Department Deployment: Integrating Quality Improvement into Day-to-Day Management," *The Quality Letter*, Vol. 6, No. 6, July–August 1994, pp. 31-39.

Galpin, Timothy. "Connecting Culture to Organizational Change," *HR Magazine*, Vol. 41, No. 3, March 1996, pp. 84-90.

Griffith, John R. *The Well Managed Health Care Organization*. Ann Arbor, MI: Health Administration Press, 1995.

Grundy, Tony. *Breakthrough Strategies for Growth*. London: Pitman, 1995.

Gupta, Mahesh and Vickie S. Campbell. "The Cost of Quality," *Production and Inventory Management Journal*, Vol. 36, No. 3, 1995, pp. 43-49.

Hayes, John. "After the Weeding: Avoiding Post-Merger Pitfalls," *The Bankers Magazine*, Vol. 179, No. 3, May/June 1996, pp. 35-39.

Heilig, Steve. "The Team Approach to Change," *Healthcare Forum Journal*, Vol. 33, No. 4, July–August 1990, pp. 19-22.

Iamai, Masaaki. *Kaizen: the Key to Japanese Competitive Success*. New York: Random House, 1986.

James, Brent C. *Quality Management for Health Care Delivery—Quality Measurement and Management Project, 7*. The Hospital Research and Educational Trust, 1989.

Joint Commission on Accreditation of Healthcare Organizations (JCAHO). *1996 Comprehensive Manual for Hospitals*. Chicago: JCAHO, 1995.

Juran, J. M. *Juran on Leadership for Quality*. New York: The Free Press, 1989.

————. "The Quality Trilogy," *Quality Progress*, Vol. 19, No. 8, August 1986, pp. 19-24.

————. and Frank M. Gryna. *Quality Planning and Analysis*, 3rd ed. New York: McGraw-Hill, 1993.

————. *Juran's Quality Control Handbook*. 4th ed. New York: McGraw-Hill, 1988.

Kaluzny, Arnold D., Curtis P. McLaughlin, and David Kibbe. "Quality Improvement: Beyond the Institution," *Hospital and Health Services Administration*, Vol. 40, No. 1, Spring 1995, pp. 172-188.

Kantor, Rosabeth Moss. "Mastering Change." in Chawla and Renesch, eds., *Learning Organizations: Developing Culture for Tomorrow's Workplace*. Portland, OR: Productivity Press, 1995.

Kaplan, Robert S. and David P. Norton. "Using the Balanced Scorecard as a Strategic Management System." *Harvard Business Review*, Vol. 74, No. 1, January–February 1996.

Kaufman, Roger. "Strategic Planning and Thinking: Alternative Views," *Performance & Instruction*, Vol. 29, No. 7, September 1990, pp. 1-7.

Kerr, Steven. "On the Folly of Rewarding A, While Hoping for B," *Academy of Management Executives*, Vol. 9, No. 1, February 1995, pp. 7-14.

Kessler, Sheila. *Total Quality Service*. Milwaukee: ASQC Quality Press, 1995.

Knaus, William P., Elizabeth A. Draper, Douglas P. Wagner, and Jack E. Zimmerman. "An Evaluation of Outcomes from Intensive Care in Major Medical Centers," *Annuals of Internal Medicine*, Vol. 104, March 1986, pp. 410-418.

Kunen, James. "The New Hands-Off Nursing," *Time*, September 30, 1996, p. 57.

Leebov, Wendy and Gail Scott. *Service Quality Improvement: The Customer Satisfaction Strategy for Health Care*. Chicago: American Hospital Publishing, 1994.

Lewin, Kurt. *Field Theory in Social Science*. New York: Harper & Row, 1951.

Luke, Roice D. and James W. Begun. "Strategy Making in Health Care Organizations," in Stephen M. Shortell and Arnold D. Kaluzny, *Health Care Management: Organization Design and Behavior*, 3rd ed. Albany, NY: Delmar Publishers, Inc., 1994.

Magnusson, Paul and Keith Hammonds. "Health Care: The Quest for Quality," *Business Week*, April 8, 1996, pp. 104-106.

Marullo, Geraldine. "Hospitals Putting Profit Margins Ahead of High-Quality Nursing Care," *Modern Healthcare*, Vol. 25, No. 6, February 6, 1995, p. 32.

Meyer, Christopher. "How the Right Measures Help Teams Excel," *Harvard Business Review*, Vol. 72, No. 3, May–June, 1994, pp. 95-103.

Migliore, Henry R. and Joe B. Gunn. "Strategic Planning/Management by Objectives," *Hospital Topics*, Vol. 73, No. 3, Summer 1995, pp. 26-32.

Morrissey, John. "N.H. Hospitals to Study Impact of Medical Care," *Modern Healthcare*, Vol. 26, No. 18, April 29, 1996, pp. 64-65.

National Committee for Quality Assurance (NCQA). *Standards for the Accreditation of Managed Care Organizations.* Washington, D.C., 1994.

———. *Health Plan Employer Data and Information Set (HEDIS) and User's Manual, Version 2.0.* Washington, D.C., 1993.

National Institute of Standards and Technology (NIST). *Malcolm Baldrige National Quality Award, Health Care Pilot Criteria.* Gaithersburg, MD: NIST, 1995.

Nelson, Bob. *1001 Ways to Reward Employees.* New York: Workman Publishing Co., 1994.

Pena, Jesus J., Alden N. Haffner, Bernard Rosen, and Donald W. Light. *Hospital Quality Assurance: Risk Management and Program Evaluation.* Rockville, MD: Aspen, 1984.

Peters, Thomas J. and Robert H. Waterman. *In Search of Excellence.* New York: Harper & Row, 1982.

——— and Nancy Austin. *A Passion for Excellence.* New York: Warner Books, 1985.

Plsek, Paul E. "Techniques for Managing Quality," *Hospital and Health Services Administration*, Vol. 40, No. 1, Spring 1995, pp. 50-79.

Reed, Richard, David J. Lemak, and Joseph C. Montgomery. "Beyond Process: TQM Content and Firm Performance," *Academy of Management Review*, Vol. 21, No. 1, 1996, pp. 173-202.

Research Triangle Institute. "Design of a Survey to Monitor Consumers' Access to Care, Use of Health Services, Health Outcomes, and Patient Satisfaction," *1996 Medical Quality Management Sourcebook*. New York: Faulkner & Gray, 1996.

Ruback, Laura. "Downsizing: How Quality is Affected as Companies Shrink," *Quality Progress*, April 1995, pp. 23-28.

Rubin, Rita and Katherine T. Beddingfield. "Rating the HMOs," *U.S. News and World Report*, September 2, 1996, pp. 52-63.

Schein, Edgar H. *Process Consultation: Its Role in Organization Development*, Vol. I, 2nd Ed. Reading, MA: Addison-Wesley, 1988.

———. *Organizational Culture and Leadership*. San Francisco: Jossey-Bass, 1992.

Schmidt, Warren H. and Jerome P. Finnigan. *The Race without a Finish Line*. San Francisco: Jossey-Bass, 1992.

Senge, Peter M. *The Fifth Discipline: The Art and Practice of the Learning Organization*. New York: Doubleday, 1990.

———, Charlotte Roberts, Richard B. Ross, Bryan J. Smith, and Art Kleiner. *The Fifth Discipline Handbook*. New York: Doubleday, 1994.

Sheridan, Bruce M. *Policy Deployment: The TQM Approach to Long-Range Planning*. Milwaukee: ASQC, 1993.

Shoemaker, Paul J.H. "Scenario Planning: A Tool for Strategic Thinking," *Sloan Management Review*, Vol. 36, No. 2, Winter 1995, pp. 25-40.

Shortell, Stephen M., Daniel Z. Levin, James L. O'Brien, and Edward F.X. Hughes. "Assessing the Evidence of CQI: Is the Glass Empty or Half Full," *Hospital and Health Services Administration,* Vol. 40, No. 1, Spring 1995, pp. 4-24.

————. Robin R. Gillies, David A. Anderson, Karen Morgan Erickson, and John B. Mitchell. *Remaking Health Care in America; Building Organized Delivery Systems.* San Francisco: Jossey-Bass, 1996.

"Strategize, Survive, Succeed," *Bank Management,* Vol. 70, No. 4, July/August 1994, pp. 8-12.

Tally, Dorsey J. *Total Quality Management Performance and Cost Measures: The Strategy for Economic Survival.* Milwaukee: ASQC Quality Press, 1991.

Taylor, Michael J., Rochelle W. Porper, and Salima Manji. "The Impact of Horizontal Mergers and Acquisitions on Cost and Quality in Health Care," *Employee Benefits Journal,* Vol. 20, No. 4, December 1995, pp. 16-19.

Thompson, Arthur A. and A.J. Strickland III. *Strategic Management.* Chicago: Irwin Professional Publishers, 1995.

Ulschak, Francis L. and Sharon M. SnowAntle. *Team Architecture: The Manager's Guide to Designing Effective Work Teams.* Ann Arbor, MI: Health Administration Press, 1995.

Vaill, Peter B. *Learning as a Way of Being.* San Francisco: Jossey-Bass, 1996.

————. *Managing as a Performing Art.* San Francisco: Jossey-Bass, 1989.

Veney, James E. and Arnold D. Kaluzny. *Evaluation and Decision Making for Health Services,* 2nd Ed. Ann Arbor, MI: Health Administration Press, 1991.

Walton, Mary. *Deming Management at Work.* New York: Putnam, 1991.

Ware, John E. Jr., Martha S. Bayliss, William H. Rogers, Mark Kosinski, and Alvin R. Tarlov. "Differences in 4-Year Health Outcomes for Elderly and Poor, Chronically Ill Patients Treated in HMO and Fee-for-Service Systems," *Journal of the American Medical Association,* Vol. 276, No. 13, October 2, 1996, pp. 1039-1047.

Whiteley, Richard C. *The Customer Driven Company.* Reading, MA: Addison-Wesley, 1991.

———— and Diane Hessan. *Customer Centered Growth: Five Proven Strategies for Building Competitive Advantage.* Reading, MA: Addison-Wesley, 1996.

Zangwill, Willard I. "Ten Mistakes CEOs Make About Quality," *Quality Progress,* Vol. 27, No. 6, June 1994, pp. 43-48.

Zelman, Walter A. "Price, Quality, and Barriers to Integration," *Frontiers of Health Services Management,* Vol. 13, No. 1, Fall 1996, pp. 43-45.

INDEX

Accreditation, 25
Acquisitions. *See* Mergers and
    acquisitions
Action plans, 14
Action Research/Organization
    Development Model, 10-16
Activity network diagramming, 103
Affinity diagrams, 46, 47, 48, 137,
    143, 172
Analysis methods, 9-10
Assessment phase, 13-14, 17-36
    approaches and tools, 20-22
    key customers, 35, 181
    mission, vision, guiding principles
      statements, 17-20, 35, 180
    models, 9, 30-33
    at Optima Health, 109-11
    philosophy, 33-34, 179-80
    staff, 73
    stakeholder analysis, 22-24
    summary/roadmap, 33-36
    See also External assessment;
      Internal assessment

Baldrige Award Health Care Pilot
    Criteria Framework, 5, 9, 30-31,
    33, 41, 119
Banking industry, 101-2
Barker, Joel, 47
Benchmarks (success measures), 10,
    14, 15-16, 105, 173
    key factors, 48, 57-58, 184-85

Brainstorming, 13, 48, 172
Budget
    capital and expense allocations,
    133-34
    cost-effective, 88-89, 173
    cost reduction, 99
    establishment of, 52-53, 60

Capozzalo, Gail, 7, 123, 136
Case examples, 107-50
    Optima Health, 107-23
    Sisters of Charity, 123-37
    Walter Reed Army Medical
      Center, 138-50
Catch-ball, 8, 55, 78, 136, 137, 182
Catholic Medical Center
    (Manchester, N.H.), 107, 121, 122
Cause-effect diagrams, 8
Change
    agents of, 155
    management of, 100, 101
    model of, 63-65
Chaufournier, Roger, 103
Climate and Readiness Survey, 33
Clinical outcome standards, 10
Columbia/HCA (Louisville, Ky.), 104
Commitment, 9, 136, 156-57
Communication, 51, 53-55, 73, 100,
    159
    transfer of learning, 95
Community resources and needs, 24
Competition, 25

203

Also available from Quality Resources ...

Quality-Centered Strategic Planning: A Step-by-Step Guide
John R. Dew, Ed.D.
222 pp., 1997, Item No. 76308X, hardcover

The Baldrige Workbook for Healthcare
Donald C. Fisher, Ph.D., and Bryan P. Simmons, M.D.
288 pp., 1996, Item No. 763136, paperback

Quality Assessment for Healthcare: A Baldrige-Based Handbook
Ned Barber, Ph.D.
204 pp., 1996, Item No. 763055, paperback

Measuring Quality Improvement in Healthcare: A Guide to Statistical
Process Control Applications
Raymond G. Carey, Ph.D., and Robert C. Lloyd, Ph.D.
208 pp., 1995, Item No. 762938, paperback

Healthcare Redesign Tools and Techniques
Jean Ann Larson
220 pp. (est.), 1997, Item No. 763225, hardcover

Value-Based Cost Management for Healthcare: Linking Costs to Quality and
Delivery
Kicab Castaneda-Mendez
189 pp., 1996, Item No. 763047, hardcover

A CQI System for Healthcare: How the Williamsport Hospital Brings
Quality to Life
Tim Mannello
318 pp., 1995, Item No. 762903, hardcover

For additional information on any of the above titles, call 800-247-8519.

Quality Resources, 902 Broadway, New York, NY 10010